The Ageless Brain

for Seniors®

**1,001 Secrets to Keep Your Brain Young,
Your Memory Sharp,
and Your Mind Healthy**

Publisher's Note

This book is intended for general information only. It does not constitute medical, legal, or financial advice or practice. The editors of FC&A have taken careful measures to ensure the accuracy and usefulness of the information in this book. While every attempt has been made to ensure accuracy, errors may occur. Some websites, addresses, and telephone numbers may have changed since printing. We cannot guarantee the safety or effectiveness of any advice or treatments mentioned. Readers are urged to consult with their professional financial advisors, lawyers, and health care professionals before making any changes.

Any health information in this book is for information only and is not intended to be a medical guide for self-treatment. It does not constitute medical advice and should not be construed as such or used in place of your doctor's medical advice. Readers are urged to consult with their health care professionals before undertaking therapies suggested by the information in this book, keeping in mind that errors in the text may occur as in all publications and that new findings may supersede older information.

The publisher and editors disclaim all liability (including any injuries, damages, or losses) resulting from the use of the information in this book.

The Lord will keep you from all harm — he will watch over your life; the Lord will watch over your coming and going both now and forevermore.
— *Psalm 121:7-8 (NIV)*

FC&A Medical Publishing®
103 Clover Green
Peachtree City, GA 30269
www.fca.com

Produced by the staff of FC&A
ISBN 978-1-935574-79-8

Table of contents

Aerobic exercise

Focus on fitness to keep your brain on track

Picture this. It's the 1980s. You're dressed in the latest workout garb. A leotard and legwarmers, maybe. You slide a tape into your VCR to start "Sweating to the Oldies."

Back then you were just trying to be more physically fit, but now — decades later — experts know you were on the right road to brain fitness, too. Keeping your brain sharp may be as simple as doing some aerobic activity even after you turn 70.

Build up brain volume with a workout. Aerobic exercise increases the circulation of oxygen through your blood and gets your breathing rate up. It's great for your body and your brain.

A healthy prefrontal cortex, PFC in brain-surgeon jargon, is important for a good memory. And the more matter you have there, the better off you are. In one study, folks participated in either a six-month aerobic exercise program or a program that featured stretching and toning exercises. The aerobic exercisers showed an increase in gray and white matter where it counts, in the PFC.

Bike your way to a better memory. Do you know the first signs of AD? You might be surprised by the answers.

* memory loss that disrupts daily life
* difficulty solving problems
* confusion about time and place
* problems with reading and judging distances
* difficulty with speaking or writing

- withdrawal from activities
- changes in mood

But the good news? You can slow AD's progress. Experts believe aerobic exercise may be the ticket for improving brain function, and it may even slow cognitive decline in people with AD. A small study of senior men with AD found that three sessions per week on an exercise bike was enough to improve participants' attention, memory, and language skills in just three months.

> Exercise beefs up your brain — that's a fact. But it also gives you a leg up on staying healthy. Exercise burns calories, helps lower blood pressure and cholesterol, eases symptoms of depression, and can kick diabetes to the curb. Start with low-impact aerobics and go slow. Check with your doctor before you start.

Perchance to dream: Exercise brings on sweet slumber

Catch 40 winks. Take a snooze. Hit the sack. All fun ways to say "go to sleep." Easy to say, but sometimes hard to do. Especially for older adults. In fact, 44% of seniors suffer from insomnia.

Don't become a slumber stat. Read on to find out how exercise can put an end to your search for a good night's sleep.

Benjamin Franklin said, "Fatigue is the best pillow." And, as usual, old Ben was right on the money. Studies show that adults with insomnia fall asleep more quickly, sleep longer, and report better sleep quality after beginning a long-term exercise program.

So why does physical activity help? Good question. Exercise causes your body temperature to rise, and experts believe the drop that follows may help you fall asleep more easily. Being active also eases the symptoms of anxiety and depression, two conditions often linked to insomnia.

Finally, some people suffer from insomnia because their internal body clock — also known as circadian rhythm — isn't working properly. Researchers believe exercise helps get your sleep-wake cycle back on track.

Power up your body to perk up your brain

You already know that sitting around too much — at a desk, say, or in front of the TV — increases your risk of developing unhealthy conditions like obesity. Need another reason to get up? New research says middle-aged and older adults who spend extended periods of time sitting may be more likely to develop memory problems.

A small study of folks between the ages of 45 and 75 found that those who reported sitting the most hours each day also had the most thinning in an area of the brain called the medial temporal lobe. Brain thinning can be an early sign of dementia.

The scientists say more research is needed. But, they add, reducing the amount of time spent in a chair may help improve the brain health of people at risk for Alzheimer's disease.

Boost your get-up-and-go with these easy tips

Exercise helps trigger the release of chemicals in your brain that lift your mood, relieve stress, and improve your sleep. But getting motivated to work out can be, well, quite a workout. These simple suggestions will help you take that first step. And another. And another. You get the idea.

- Set realistic goals. If you're just starting out, you might try walking down the block and back, or simply do stretches while watching TV.

- Be consistent. Exercise at the same time each day.

- Don't be hard on yourself if you miss a session. The important thing is to get back on track.

- Keep a log of your progress so you can see how much you've accomplished.

- Use a pedometer to count your steps.

- Make it fun. Walk with a friend or join an exercise class.

- Reward yourself for meeting your goals.

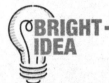

BRIGHT IDEA

3 fun ways to ramp up your exercise routine

You've probably heard about the multi-sport National Senior Games, an Olympics-style competition for folks age 50 and over. Well, in 2019 Mary Crusius took home the gold for her power-house performance on the pickleball court. That's nice, you might say. But Mary aced the match at the ripe young age of 91.

Read on to learn more about pickleball and other fabulous ways to work out at any age.

Get in tiptop shape with pickleball. Imagine a mashup of tennis, badminton, and pingpong. How fun! No wonder this game is gaining popularity with seniors everywhere. And it's a heart-healthy aerobic exercise that boosts your hand-eye coordination but isn't too hard on your body. You don't need expensive equipment — paddles cost as little as $12. Check online at *places2play.org* to find pickleball leagues near you.

Cycle up for more brainpower. Just 10 minutes of aerobic activity — like riding a stationary bike — can perk up the parts of the brain that help you focus and solve problems. But do you choose the recumbent or upright style? If you're look-ing for comfort, recumbent is the one for you. The chair-like seat supports your back, and the reclined position keeps you from straining.

Improve flexibility with a water workout. Want to take pressure off your aching joints? Try water aerobics. It gets an A-plus when it comes to improving your flexibility and easing lower back pain. Contact your local public pools, gyms, and recreation centers for class schedules.

Anti-inflammatory diet

Tame the flame to upgrade your brain

What's painful, swollen, and red all over? Damaged tissue that has become inflamed. When you nick yourself with a knife or stub your toe, white blood cells — your immune system's first responders — rush in to ward off infection and repair damaged tissue.

Acute inflammation is a healthy and short-lived immune response that aids in recovery. But a constant state of inflammation — what occurs when your immune system fails to eliminate an infectious organism, for example — can prompt those same white blood cells to attack healthy tissue. In fact, chronic inflammation can do a number on your noggin. Luckily, what you put on your plate can turn the tide.

Save your thinking skills with antioxidants A study in the *Journal of Psychosomatic Research* shows that higher levels of inflammation can negatively affect executive functioning. Those are the skills you need for things like flexible thinking, which allows you to solve a problem in more than one way. Trouble with executive functioning can make it harder to manage your emotions, focus, and follow directions.

Fortunately, adding antioxidants to your diet may ward off inflammation of the brain, a condition associated with cognitive decline and Alzheimer's disease (AD). Antioxidants also neutralize or remove free radicals — unstable molecules that damage cells and may contribute to the formation of plaques found in the brains of people with AD.

You can get the antioxidants you need from fruits and vegetables like blueberries, strawberries, kale, red cabbage, and artichokes.

Drop inflammatory foods to retain brain health. Too much inflammation is no joke — it can even affect the size of your brain. A study published in *Neurology* found that people with elevated levels of inflammation at midlife were more likely to have smaller brain volumes decades later. They were also more likely to experience reduced episodic memory in their senior years.

What's episodic memory? It's your unique recall of a specific event, like your first day at a new job or where you were when your first grandchild was born.

But you may be able to protect your brain by watching what you eat. A large study found that diets high in fried foods and red and processed meats — but low in whole grains — were linked to higher levels of inflammation and faster cognitive decline.

Why is this combo, which is often found in Western diets, bad for your brain? Such diets tend to be high in unhealthy fats that increase your risk of inflammation. Moreover, they often lack the inflammation-fighting antioxidants found in unrefined grains, fruits, and vegetables.

It's easy to find a cut-and-dried way to stick to anti-inflammatory foods. The Mediterranean and DASH diets both feature foods that are high in inflammation-busting omega-3 fatty acids and antioxidants. Read about the other benefits of these food plans later in this book.

Top conditions caused by inflammation (and how to stop them at the source)

In 1985, residents of a houseboat community in Sausalito, California were shocked to discover that the source of an obnoxious humming noise on summer nights was none other than the singing toadfish. The unknown cause of the ruckus led to many a sleepless night.

You, on the other hand, may have a different kind of hidden problem that causes even bigger issues. When chronic inflammation lurks under the surface, it can wreak all kinds of havoc.

For the people of Sausalito, earplugs are the only solution. But you have options when it comes to silencing inflammation.

Inflammation plays a lead role in many conditions. You already know that inflammation in the brain is linked to cognitive decline and Alzheimer's disease. But chronic inflammation can also lead to numerous other heath conditions that negatively impact how well your brain works.

• Diabetes. Everyone with diabetes is in the same boat when it comes to inflammation. Although the causes and risk factors of type 1 and type 2 diabetes are different, chronic inflammation is associated with both types of this disease.

• Heart disease. The immune system cells that cause inflammation can injure your blood vessels and add to the buildup of fatty deposits in arteries. This plaque accumulation can lead to artery blockage and cause a heart attack.

• Arthritis. In rheumatoid arthritis, your body's immune system attacks the lining that encloses your joints. The lining — dubbed the synovial membrane — becomes swollen and inflamed. The condition can damage the cartilage and bone in your joints.

• Cancer. Your immune system cells normally hunt down and devour damaged cells that can become cancerous. But chronic inflammation can create an environment that allows cancer cells to develop into a tumor. It may even hurt how well your body responds to therapy.

Kick inflammation instigators to the curb. Nixing inflammatory foods from your diet is a great way to stay healthy. Why not remove these other common causes of inflammation from your life?

• excess body weight   • lack of exercise

• stress   • smoking

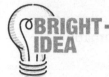

Eat this, not that:
Easy food sensitivity swaps

No fried food? No problem. Prepare to be amazed by the variety anti-inflammatory diets offer. You may feel like you're cutting out a lot, but eating an abundance of fresh foods is a tasty way to protect your body. Try these simple meal swaps to save yourself from chronic inflammation.

- Trade red and processed meat for other protein sources. You may miss burgers and hot dogs at first, but that doesn't mean you're out of options. Fatty fish like salmon and tuna have lots of protein. And they're loaded with inflammation-busting omega-3 fatty acids to boot. Sprinkle almonds and walnuts onto high-quality yogurt for an extra punch of protein. Soy beans are an especially good source of this important nutrient.

- Skip unhealthy fats like margarine, shortening, and lard when possible. And use extra-virgin olive oil instead of safflower and sunflower oils.

- Limit refined carbohydrates by cutting down on white bread and white rice. Whole grains, like those found in brown rice and bulgur wheat, are better for you. Can't imagine dropping pasta? Spaghetti squash is a veggie alternative you can eat guilt-free.

- Avoid sugary-sweet drinks like soda. Choose water instead. If you're looking for something more flavorful, brew a tasty pot of green or oolong tea.

- Ditch processed foods and add nutrient-rich fresh fare in their place. Fruits like strawberries, blueberries, and oranges are great choices. Spinach, kale, and collards make for excellent veggie options.

Apples

Bolster brain health with nature's super snack

Pull out that apple juice you keep in the fridge for the grandkids, and pour yourself a glass. Or two. Because according to studies, apples and apple juice have what it takes to juice up your brain.

Apple juice keeps Alzheimer's disease (AD) at bay. Ever heard of acetylcholine? Probably not. But it's famous in the world of AD researchers. Scientists have discovered that apple juice may actually prevent the breakdown of acetylcholine in your body. That's important because people with AD often have low levels of this neurotransmitter — a chemical that nerve cells release to communicate with each other — in their brains.

In a monthlong animal study, researchers compared two groups of mice that were genetically programmed to develop AD. They found the mice that drank water mixed with apple juice concentrate had higher levels of acetylcholine in their brains compared with mice that drank plain water. The mice that were given the apple juice also performed significantly better on maze memory tests compared with the other mice.

A very good sign. The researchers say apple juice may have a one-of-a-kind mix of antioxidants — substances that can prevent or slow damage to cells — that prevents declines in acetylcholine levels in the brain.

The amount of apple juice given to the one group of mice was comparable to drinking two 8-ounce glasses, or eating two to three apples, each day.

Fisetin fights to keep your brain healthy. Fisetin is a flavonoid — a plant chemical — that researchers say shows great promise in protecting the brain from dementia, memory loss, and AD. Fisetin is found in many of your favorite fruits and vegetables, like apples. Strawberries, onions, and tomatoes are also good sources.

In a separate study of mice that were genetically programmed to develop AD, researchers fed some of the animals water mixed with fisetin. The remaining mice drank plain water. Nine months later, the mice given water with fisetin remained healthy. And those who drank the plain water? They began showing signs of cognitive decline.

Follow the apple's star to healthy eating. Cut an apple across the middle. Look inside, and you'll find a five-pointed star. Surprise! What you're seeing are five seed pockets, or carpels. The health of the apple tree and the variety of apple determine the amount of seeds in each carpel.

The researchers say fisetin has anti-inflammatory properties and the ability to reduce oxidative stress, a process in the body that damages cells, proteins, and DNA. Oxidative stress may also play a role in the development of AD.

Enjoy an apple or a cool glass of apple juice every day. And keep those doctors far, far away.

Benefits by the bushel: How about them apples?

You've probably heard this oldie-but-goodie proverb a thousand times, but just not in these words. Consume one of these fruits, the *Malus domestica*, every 24 hours, and physicians will steer clear of your premises. Figured it out yet? An apple a day keeps the doctor away, of course.

You already know apples may help fight Alzheimer's disease, but read on to find out all the other things this luscious fruit can do for you.

- Arthritis. Quercetin, a powerful antioxidant found in apple peels, has been shown to relieve symptoms of early morning stiffness in people with rheumatoid arthritis.

- Bones. Apples contain nutrients including vitamin C, vitamin K, potassium, and magnesium that are necessary for bone health.

- Constipation. Apple pectin is a soluble fiber that helps speed up the movement of stool through the intestines. Just two daily servings of fiber-rich fruits like apples promotes regularity.

- Diarrhea. The same apple pectin that relieves constipation also helps with diarrhea. Apple pectin bulks up the stool to relieve diarrhea symptoms.

- Eyes. Researchers believe quercetin also shows great promise in the treatment of ocular surface diseases like dry eye, a condition that causes your eyes to feel gritty or scratchy. Advanced dry eye may hurt the surface of your eyes and even damage your vision.

- Cholesterol. Have high cholesterol? Studies show that eating two apples a day can reduce total cholesterol and LDL, the bad kind of cholesterol. That apple pectin at work again. Polyphenols — healthy compounds found in plant-based foods — may also play a role.

- Gingivitis. Resveratrol is a polyphenol found in foods like peanuts, berries, and — you guessed it — apples. Its anti-inflammatory and antioxidant properties make resveratrol a natural for keeping teeth and gums healthy. Apples are also a good source of vitamin C, which helps slow the progression of — and even prevent — periodontal disease.

- Kidneys. Your kidneys help regulate the amount of potassium in your body. But if your kidneys are unhealthy, you might need to avoid foods that have high amounts of this mineral. Apples are low in potassium, so they're a good choice for your diet plan. And the pectin in apples may also lower your risk of high blood sugar, which can damage your kidneys.

- Heart. This time it's the apple skin that gets all the glory. In one study, researchers believe the flavonoids in apple peels may have helped reduce blood pressure and improve endothelial function — how well blood vessels work — in people at risk for cardiovascular disease.

So as you can see, just about every part of you will say thank you after you eat this disease-fighting fruit.

BRIGHT IDEA

Pesticides bugging you?
Apples come clean with these easy tips

Don't let pesticides get under your skin. Believe it or not, the United States Department of Agriculture (USDA) has found pesticide residue on the produce you eat every day. Yep, even on your favorite apples. In fact, more than 90% of tested apples turned up positive for the residue of at least two or more pesticides.

Follow these tips to get your apples clean as a whistle.

- Go organic. Buying organic fruits and veggies is the safest way avoid to pesticides. That's because organic produce isn't exposed to man-made pesticides.

- Clean the right way. Wash all fruit and vegetables when you get home from the store by rubbing them under running water. The longer pesticides stay on your food, the deeper they're absorbed.

- Go the extra mile. For extra protection, place your apples and other produce in a solution of 1 teaspoon of baking soda and 2 cups of water. Soak for at least two minutes. Have some extra time? Researchers found that soaking apples in water and baking soda for 12 to 15 minutes was the best way to get rid of all the pesticides used in the study.

- Turn on the faucet. Rinse thoroughly in tap water before eating.

Aromatherapy

Sniff your way to a sharper memory

You've probably noticed that your sense of smell can trigger powerful, long-forgotten memories. A whiff of freshly baked bread can whisk you back to, say, Sunday meals at Grandma's.

So how does your nose transport you back in time? Your sense of smell activates a part of your brain called the limbic system that deals with memories and emotions. It's one of the reasons researchers believe aromatherapy — the therapeutic use of scented plant- and flower-based essential oils — can help keep your memory sharp. Here are three herbs you won't forget.

Rosemary revs up recall. You may instinctively brush a leaf from your hair if it blows there on a windy day. The ancient Greeks had a different perspective — at least when it comes to rosemary. Students used to purposefully stick a sprig of this herb in their hair to improve memory and concentration during exams.

So were they on to something? It seems so, according to researchers who tested 66 people in either a rosemary-scented room or one with no aroma. They found that the participants who inhaled the rosemary performed better on prospective memory tests. That's the kind of memory you need to perform a future activity, like remembering to pick up groceries on your way home or attend a birthday party next week.

In a separate study, exposure to rosemary aroma appears to have boosted participants' ability to subtract numbers quickly and accurately.

Unlock memories with lavender. Surprise — along with rosemary, lavender is actually part of the mint family. Here's something else unexpected. Researchers found that the soothing scent of lavender improved the working memory of people after they took a stressful test.

Your working memory helps you store and process information over the short term. You use this type of memory, for example, when you multiply numbers without scratch paper.

Just sniffing three drops of diluted lavender oil was enough to get a boost from the purple plant.

Peppermint peps up recollection. You may have heard peppermint tea can perk you up. But that's not this herb's only claim to fame. Research published in the *American Journal of Plant Sciences* found that inhaling peppermint oil boosts memory.

One hundred participants were randomly assigned to wear a patch infused with peppermint oil or a scentless patch. After six hours they were tested on things like word recall, prospective memory, and how many words beginning with the letter "s" they could write down in one minute. The researchers found that the peppermint oil group performed better on the tests, and even showed signs of being more alert and attentive.

A separate study found that four drops of the essential oil diffused across a room significantly improved prospective memory.

Soothing scents: Exhale your anxieties with aromatherapy

Feeling stressed? Spritzing some essential oils around the room may be all you need to banish your anxiety — without the side effects of common medications.

Some mood meds come with a side order of headaches, drowsiness, sleep woes, and more. But studies show aromatherapy can work wonders without those unpleasant symptoms. That's one reason experts say essential oils may be a good alternative or complementary treatment. Talk to your doctor about including one of these oils as part of your game plan.

Lavender lifts your worries. Just the idea of being hospitalized is enough to make anybody anxious. But a two-day study of 60 intensive-care patients suggests that a little purple flower called lavender naturally lowers the anxiety that comes with a stressful hospital stay.

According to the research, half of the participants deeply inhaled the aroma of lavender essential oils a total of 10 times before going to sleep. A nearby diffuser continued to spread the lavender scent throughout the night. The other half of patients didn't have any aromatherapy.

Compared with the control group, the people who received the lavender treatment showed improvements in their blood pressure, heart rate, and sleep quality — three conditions often negatively affected by stress and anxiety. Other studies, meanwhile, attest to lavender's ability to calm anxiety symptoms without negative side effects.

> Essential oils come in a wide variety. So if one isn't right for you — maybe you just don't like the scent — chances are you'll find another that fits the bill. Along with lavender and bergamot, oils that lower stress and anxiety levels include ylang-ylang, clary sage, and chamomile.

Breathe in bergamot to ease stress. You may recognize this fragrant citrus fruit — it's about the size of an orange with a thin yellow or green rind — as an ingredient in your Earl Grey tea. But bergamot is more than a flavor booster.

A Taiwanese study of people awaiting outpatient surgery found that 30 minutes of aromatherapy with bergamot essential oils eased anxiety better than water vapor. It didn't matter whether they had surgery before or not.

The researchers aren't exactly sure why, but believe the results may have something to do with bergamot's ability to trigger the release of amino acids that aid in the passage of messages between nerve cells.

BRIGHT IDEA

Stay safe buying and using essential oils

Aromatherapy is more than simply finding a nice scent and taking it home. Picking the best quality oil and using it correctly are key when it comes to improving your health.

Be a savvy shopper and buy essential oils in dark bottles. The tinted glass helps to keep the oil from deteriorating. Check the label's Latin name to make sure it matches what you're looking for.

Several species of lavender exist — *Lavandula angustifolia* and *Lavandula latifolia*, for example — and you want to get the oil best suited to your needs.

Be sure you're buying 100% pure essential oil by looking at the purity statement. And keep an eye out for a quality seal, such as GRAS-certified (generally recognized as safe) or USP (U.S. Pharmacopeia). Be sure to keep the container tightly closed in a cool location to ward off heat, light, and oxygen.

Lots of people inhale essential oils by diffusing them in a room. Want to go the topical route? Follow these safety tips to avoid an allergic reaction.

- Dilute with a carrier oil to protect your skin from irritation.

- Test for an allergic reaction on a small patch of skin.

- Never dab essential oils around your eyes or on broken skin.

- Don't apply to the same spot every day.

- Skip putting citrus oils on your skin.

Check with your doctor before using essential oils because they can worsen symptoms of underlying health conditions and interact with some medications. And remember that essential oils can be toxic if swallowed.

Art therapy

Preserve your memory through art

Lonni Sue Johnson was a respected artist when she developed inflammation of the brain and permanently lost her memory. What has helped her in her journey to recovery? She creates pictures of words and images that reinforce her long-term memory of concepts and processes. But art doesn't just help your brain heal. As recent studies have shown, it can protect your noggin in more ways than one.

Creating art wards off memory loss. Can a lump of clay or dabs of paint help keep your brain young? Research suggests so.

According to a study in the journal *Neurology*, seniors who engaged in the arts — painting, drawing, or sculpting, for example — during their middle and later years were 73% less likely to develop mild cognitive impairment (MCI) over four years than those who didn't create art. MCI is the stage between the normal decline in memory, language, and thinking that comes with aging and the serious decline that comes with dementia.

Prefer crafts like sewing, quilting, or woodworking over art? The scientists found that older folks who crafted in their middle and

Say cheese! Snap those campy grins. You enjoy the moment more when you see it through the camera lens, according to researchers at the University of Southern California. Even thinking about taking a picture helps you savor the occasion because you feel more engaged in it.

senior years were 45% less likely to develop MCI over four years compared with those who didn't craft. The researchers believe keeping your mind actively engaged in arts and crafts protects your brain's nerve cells from dying off and may even prompt new ones to grow.

Gallery crawls boost recall. You don't have to create your own masterpiece to benefit from art. That's according to a small study of older adults with dementia who participated in a six-week art appreciation program at the National Gallery of Australia. Educators presented them with three to four works each week. The seniors learned art-related terms, talked about art, and were challenged with new ideas and cultural experiences.

At the end of the program, the seniors reported feeling less depressed. They also showed improvements in their working memory — the ability to temporarily store and manage the information needed to carry out a task — and their ability to retrieve words. But that's not all.

"Six weeks after the study, we asked participants what they remembered of the visits, and almost 50% were able to recall specific aspects of the program," says Nathan D'Cunha, lead researcher for the project at the University of Canberra.

Are you ready to be inspired? Visit art galleries and talk to others about what you see. Or look for arts and crafts programs at senior centers, public libraries, memory care centers, or hospitals. If your community isn't offering an art program, ask one of those resources to create one.

State of the art: Create more, stress less

The artist Jackson Pollock developed a unique style of painting in the 1940s. He dripped, poured, and scattered house paint across huge canvases spread out on his studio floor. One reason why? He cared more about expressing his emotions than making his pictures represent anything real.

Perhaps Pollock was on to something. Recent research suggests that communicating your feelings through art can help you manage health problems like stress and depression.

A study at Drexel University found that creating art for just 45 minutes can significantly lower levels of the stress hormone cortisol in your body. Researchers tested the amount of cortisol in the saliva of 39 adults before and after they used markers, paper, modeling clay, and collage materials to create a piece of art. Sure enough, 75% of the participants' cortisol levels dropped during the experiment.

> Feeling blue? Pull out a pencil. Research suggests just three minutes of doodling or freehand drawing can boost your mood — regardless of your skill level. Scientists believe creating art activates the part of your brain that produces feelings of reward and pleasure.

In this study, an art therapist was available if the participants needed or wanted help.

Art therapists are professionally trained counselors and artists. They use the production of art — painting, drawing, and sculpting, for example — to give voice to what troubles you. How? By helping you examine and cope with the underlying psychological or emotional messages that you communicate during the creative process.

Studies show working with an art therapist has other benefits.

- Ease pain. Control your physical pain with a pencil? You bet. Drawing as a form of art therapy can help lower your perception of pain by teaching you how to relax and not focus on your physical discomfort. It also helps you manage the anxiety that often accompanies pain.

- Ease symptoms of depression. Art therapy won't cure depression, but it can help put you on the road to recovery. That's according to a study of people with depression who were treated with 10 hourlong sessions of art therapy as part of an overall treatment plan. Those who doodled and painted and discussed their work with an art therapist showed more improvement in their symptoms than people in a control group.

BRIGHT IDEA

Draw or color your worries away

Think back to when you learned to write the alphabet. Remember leaning over your tablet, pencil in hand, fixing your attention on the lines of each letter? Did you know that focusing on lines, circles, and curves can help you relax even now? Next time you're feeling stressed, get in touch with your inner child through drawing or coloring.

Relax and refocus with abstract drawing. Just you, a pen with black ink, and a blank piece of paper — that's all you need to get an emotional boost from freehand drawing. Just be sure to give your inner perfectionist the day off. Draw what you want — any form that captures your feelings — instead of trying to create an exact likeness of, say, a bird or vase of flowers.

Create a pattern by repeating the same pen strokes. Tune in to the sound of the pen gliding across the page and breathe deeply. Not working with colors and an eraser limits distracting decisions and keeps you from worrying about "fixing" your drawing. Remember that imperfection is part of the process.

Want to know more about drawing simple, structured patterns to help you unwind? Head over to *zentangle.com*.

Melt stress away with colored pencils. Mandala coloring books are very different from the kind your grandchildren use. Full of patterns and fine lines, they can help you cope with anxiety. On stressful days, pick a mandala with a simple design. Whip out your colored pencils for 20 or 30 minutes and you will likely feel more relaxed.

Not keen on mandalas? Consider a gratitude coloring book. It provides space for journaling about the things you appreciate in life.

Aspirin

The humble aspirin may be your brain's best friend

Benjamin Franklin once famously observed that "an ounce of prevention is worth a pound of cure." You can use this strategy in your fight against dementia. How? Pick up a bottle of aspirin.

This cheap, easy-to-get home remedy pill is called a nonsteroidal anti-inflammatory drug (NSAID). You probably use aspirin and other NSAIDs like ibuprofen and naproxen to treat fever, headaches, and painful joints. But some researchers think aspirin might be the "vaccine" that prevents deadly Alzheimer's disease (AD).

Prevent Alzheimer's disease. Studies suggest that people with type 2 diabetes have a higher risk of developing AD. Possible reasons? Complications from diabetes can damage blood vessels in the brain. In addition, high blood sugar levels lead to inflammation, which may harm brain cells.

Fortunately, a large, eight-year study of people with type 2 diabetes found that those who took less than 40 milligrams (mg) of aspirin a day were less likely to develop AD than participants who didn't take aspirin regularly.

The researchers didn't provide a reason for their results. But a separate study on mice genetically engineered to develop AD suggests that aspirin helps clear out cellular waste. Researchers also believe the drug hinders the formation of plaques seen in the brains of people with AD.

Remember that evidence on aspirin's effectiveness in warding off AD is limited. Talk to your doctor if you're considering taking aspirin, as it can increase the risk of bleeding in the brain and stomach.

Defend your memory. In a two-year study that included seniors with either normal cognitive functioning or mild cognitive impairment (MCI), researchers found that the participants who took NSAIDs had better executive function skills — the ability to plan, switch focus, and remember details, for example — than the comparable control groups who didn't use this type of medication.

MCI is the stage between the normal lapses in memory, judgment, and language that occur with aging and the more serious decline that comes with dementia.

In addition, the researchers found that NSAID use was associated with higher scores on memory tests in women with normal cognitive skills. They say NSAIDs may boost these skills by slowing down the rate that you lose brain cells during normal aging.

Studies suggest that taking NSAIDs in middle age, or at least before the age of 65, brings the most brain-boosting benefits.

Get proven medicine for life-changing conditions

It sure would be great if you could prevent a heart attack, stroke, or migraine from ever happening. The best way to achieve this goal is to adopt a healthy lifestyle. But that may not be enough. People at high risk for these conditions might find low-cost relief in aspirin.

Sidestep a heart attack or stroke. Aspirin works wonders when it comes to preventing artery-blocking blood clots. That's why many people with heart disease take it regularly. But you should talk to your doctor about your risk of having a heart attack or stroke before starting aspirin therapy.

The Aspirin in Reducing Events in the Elderly project (ASPREE) suggests that taking a low-dose aspirin every day poses more risk than benefit in healthy seniors with no history of cardiovascular disease. Researchers found that rates for major cardiovascular events — including heart attacks and strokes — were similar in older adults who took a daily aspirin and those who didn't. But the aspirin takers ran a significantly higher risk of serious bleeding in their gastrointestinal tract and brain compared with seniors who didn't take aspirin each day.

Still, it's worth it to see if aspirin therapy might be helpful to you. Ask your doctor for an atherosclerotic cardiovascular disease risk (ASCVD) estimation to gauge your risk of having a heart attack or stroke.

Control migraines. Research suggests that plain old aspirin works just as well in preventing and treating migraines as more expensive medicines.

> Did you know your brain's hippocampus — its memory center — is shaped like a sea horse? Here's another fascinating fact. Researchers have found that London cab drivers have larger-than-average hippocampi. Why? Because of the workout their brains get memorizing the swiftest routes between London's 25,000 maze-like streets.

According to a report in *The American Journal of Medicine*, 900 to 1,300 milligrams (mg) of aspirin taken at the onset of symptoms is an effective treatment option for acute migraines. Researchers suggest a lower daily dose of between 81 and 325 mg as a way to prevent recurring migraines.

One reason aspirin is so effective? Its anti-inflammatory properties may help prevent the migraine-triggering dilation of blood vessels in your brain.

Prevent a major stroke — know the warning signs

Is it a ministroke or just a dizzy spell? Sometimes it's hard to tell, but knowing if you're facing a health emergency or just having a bad day could save your life.

Problems like low blood sugar, migraines, and minor seizures can mimic symptoms of a ministroke, or transient ischemic attack (TIA).

The difference is the effects of a TIA are more likely to be localized rather than widespread.

Symptoms may only last a few minutes. But instead of self-diagnosing, go to the hospital ASAP. Or call 911 if you notice any of the eight telltale symptoms that a stroke is underway or has occurred.

- sudden, severe headache
- weakness or numbness in the face, arm, or leg, especially on one side of the body
- mental confusion
- memory loss
- dizziness, drowsiness, or falls
- difficulty speaking or slurred speech
- a loss or blurring of vision
- nausea and vomiting

Afterward, your doctor may recommend taking aspirin to prevent a secondary stroke. Why? About 9 out of 10 strokes are ischemic, most often caused by a blood clot blocking an artery in the brain. Aspirin is considered an anti-platelet drug, and prevents blood cells called platelets from clumping together to form a clot. Because of this, the American Heart Association recommends people suffering an ischemic stroke receive aspirin within 24 to 48 hours of symptoms.

However, medical doctors have long feared that taking aspirin might increase the risk of bleeding or death in the 1 stroke victim out of 10 suffering the more rare hemorrhagic stroke — where a weakened artery ruptures and bleeds into the brain. Now in-depth studies that included patients with bleeding strokes who were given aspirin found this wasn't so.

A decision analysis published in the journal *Neurology* concluded aspirin treatment, given even without knowing the type of stroke, is likely to decrease the risk of a second stroke and increase the survival rate after discharge from the hospital.

And the highly respected medical analysis group, The NNT, reports that aspirin should be started as soon as possible after a stroke, since in the first 24 hours bleeding in the brain is unlikely but suffering a second ischemic stroke is relatively common.

Be sure to check with your doctor for his advice about taking aspirin for stroke or treating any serious medical emergency.

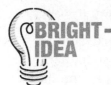

BRIGHT IDEA

Head to the pantry to reap the benefits without the risks

An organic veggie sandwich on whole-grain bread is a smart choice for any meal. Why? It's loaded with salicylic acid (SA), the active ingredient in aspirin responsible for its anti-inflammatory effects.

Fruits and veggies like blackberries, green beans, white onions, and green apples have SA. And because they're plant-based foods, they contain nutrients that appear to protect the lining of the stomach from the side effects of long-term aspirin use.

Of course you could never completely replace aspirin therapy with plant sources of SA. But Michael Greger, M.D., physician and advocate for a whole-food, plant-based diet, reports that people who eat fruits and vegetables have significantly higher levels of SA than those who don't — often enough to affect inflammation. Next time you head to the grocery, make this your short list.

Go organic. So how does a plant protect itself from bugs? It produces and stores SA in its most vulnerable parts — its roots, leaves, seeds, and skin. But plants sprayed with pesticides have lower concentrations of SA. After all, they've got man-made protection against pests. And that means less SA for you.

Spice up your palate. You'll get the highest concentrations of SA from herbs and spices like oregano, thyme, red chili powder, paprika, and turmeric. A teaspoon of cumin has roughly the same amount of SA as a baby aspirin.

Focus on whole grains. Look for breads with the 100% whole-grain stamp. They're high in SA and have 100 times more phytochemicals — healthy plant compounds that may lower your risk of disease — than white bread made with refined flour.

Memory mishaps may be your meds instead

Fuzzy thinking? Memory slipping? Slow reactions? It may not be Alzheimer's disease (AD), but an easily reversible condition instead.

A toxic reaction to prescription and over-the-counter medications can cause reversible dementia and delirium, a confused state that makes it hard to think, focus, and remember. For example, the side effects of some anticholinergic drugs used to treat conditions like depression, incontinence, and muscle spasms can impair thinking skills, particularly in older adults.

Signs and symptoms of delirium usually start abruptly and can change from day to day. On the other hand, symptoms of AD — forgetting newly learned information and having trouble following a conversation, for example — develop steadily over time.

Fortunately, you can take steps to prevent reversible dementia and delirium. Look in your medicine cabinet for 17 of the most prescribed drugs that are common causes of memory loss. You'll find them in the following table. If you're concerned about symptoms and taking any of these medications, talk to your doctor about alternatives that might be available.

Type	Drug
anticonvulsants	clonazepam, lamotrigine, lorazepam
antihistamines	azelastine, desloratadine
benzodiazepines	clorazepate, temazepam
corticosteroids	cortisone, hydrocortisone, prednisone
opiates	butorphanol, hydromorphone
tricyclic antidepressants	amoxapine
fluoroquinolone antibiotics	ciprofloxacin, levofloxacin
H2-antagonists	famotidine
anticholinergics	benztropine

Avocados

Lutein launches your brainpower above and beyond

Avocados are worth the time they take to ripen. You'll trade a hard and bitter snack for one that's soft and buttery. But one thing you don't want to turn soft is your aging brain. Luckily, this nourishing fruit keeps your mind sharp with the help of the antioxidant lutein.

Boost brain performance with this tropical fruit. Avocados make a great addition to your veggie-based smoothies. But don't let them fool you. They're actually fruits. That big pit in the middle is the only clue you need — fruits grow from flowering plants and have seeds. Vegetables, on the other hand, are the roots, stems, and leaves of plants.

Whether you call it a fruit or veggie doesn't matter when it comes to helping your brain. When you eat a slice of this creamy power-house, your brain and macula — the center part of your eye's retina — readily absorb lutein. Scientists measure the lutein in the macula because higher levels there reflect a higher concentration in your brain. And that's just what you need to think more clearly as you age.

Researchers from Tufts University set out to measure the brain benefits of avocado. The study, published in *Nutrients*, showed that healthy adults who ate a fresh avocado daily for six months increased their macular lutein levels by 25% and performed better on cognitive tests than participants who didn't eat avocados.

The avocado eaters' attention spans improved, as did their ability to temporarily store and use information. Plus their problem-solving skills got better.

Drop your dementia risk with your diet. Lutein doesn't just protect your memory today, it guards your mind's future, too. A 10-year study of French seniors found that those who had higher concentrations of lutein in their blood had a lower risk of developing dementia and Alzheimer's disease (AD).

Lutein is mainly present in parts of the brain that are vulnerable to AD and likely keeps you healthy by fighting oxidation and inflammation.

Avocados ace the case for heart disease, eyesight, and more

Avocado-colored kitchens have fallen out of fashion, but the fatty fruit that inspired them is more than a fad. From your waist to your head, avocados can help keep you fit as a fiddle.

Feel full longer. An afternoon snack may be the perfect pick-me-up, but unhealthy eating between meals can cause unwanted weight gain. And that's not good for your brain. After all, obesity can raise your risk of developing dementia. So how do you prevent demanding hunger pangs? Fill in the gap with avocado.

Just one half of this delicious fruit can keep you full for a whopping five hours. A study published in *Nutrition Journal* found that healthy but overweight adults who added half an avocado to their lunch dropped much of their desire to snack three hours later. After five hours, they still felt less hungry than usual.

Lower LDL cholesterol. Avocado toast recently became a trendy health food — and for good reason, according to researchers.

"When people incorporated one avocado a day into their diet, they had fewer small, dense LDL particles than before the diet," says Penny Kris-Etherton, distinguished professor of nutrition and co-author of a study on the health effects of avocado. All LDL is bad cholesterol, but the kind Kris-Etherton mentions is even more unhealthy. The particles had become oxidized, which could cause hardening of the arteries. "Consequently, people should consider adding avocados to their diet in a healthy way, like on whole-wheat toast or as a veggie dip."

Decreasing your levels of LDL particles can help reduce your heart disease risk. Avocados may even help control dangerous inflammation, a condition that can damage brain cells. How does this odd-looking fruit do all that? It's packed with monounsaturated fatty acids and antioxidants.

Supercharge your senses.
Sharp hearing and keen eyesight are your body's keys to the outside world, so you don't want them to fade as you age. Look no further than the tasty avocado to keep both senses working well.

This super fruit owes its powers to folate — a B vitamin that can help keep your eyes and ears healthy.

> When it comes to avocados, save your money and skip the organic options. This fruit is ranked No. 1 on the Environmental Working Group's "Clean 15" list. That means avocados are low in pesticides, which makes them among the safest produce to eat. Still, be sure to wash all fruits and veggies before eating.

- Hearing. In a study of more than 65,000 women, researchers found that those with higher amounts of folate in their diets ran a lower risk of losing their hearing. Conversely, low amounts of dietary folate were associated with a higher risk.

- Vision. Research suggests that a folate deficiency may increase your risk of age-related macular degeneration (AMD), the leading cause of blindness and low vision in older adults. Although there isn't a cure for AMD, you can decrease your chances of developing the condition by not smoking, exercising regularly, and eating a healthy diet. A good place to start? Folate-rich avocados.

Make your avocados ripe and ready

Once ripe, an avocado lasts only two or three days before turning brown and mushy. But you can extend this green fruit's shelf life by buying an unripe avocado and ripening it just before eating. Follow one of these methods to bring your snack up to snuff.

- For an avocado that's not quite ripe, slice the unpeeled fruit in half vertically and remove the pit. Wrap the two pieces separately with microwave-safe plastic wrap. Then cook the halves in the microwave for two minutes on high. Cool the wrapped avocado under cold water to stop it from cooking further.

- If your avocado is very hard, use the oven instead. Wrap your uncut fruit in tinfoil and bake it for 10 minutes at 200 degrees. Depending on how hard your avocado is, you may have to leave it in longer. Cool it in the fridge for a few minutes.

Have an avocado that's ripening too fast for you to eat? That's when your fridge comes in handy.

- Pit your avocado and coat each half of the open fruit with lemon juice or olive oil. Wrap the pieces in plastic wrap and put them in your fridge.

- Make avocado ice. Mash the fruit in a bowl and squeeze in a bit of lemon or lime juice. Spoon the mixture into an ice cube tray and freeze it. You can take the cubes out whenever you're ready and add them to a green smoothie or salad dressing.

Balance training

Stay steady: Key to long-lasting brainpower

American gymnast Simone Biles can twist, turn, and flip on a 4-inch balance beam better than anyone in the world. In fact, one of her dismounts is so spectacular it has been named the Biles in her honor. No wonder. She trains a relentless 32 hours a week to achieve her jaw-dropping results.

Maybe you're not into gymnastics, but Simone's example should inspire you to get moving for a different reason. Poor balance could signal an increased risk of dementia. But you could tip the balance in your favor by adding a little training to your daily routine.

Strive for a stable body to keep your independence. According to the *American Journal of Preventive Medicine,* as many as 45,164 serious falls that require medical treatment could be avoided each year. Fortunately, simple, no-cost exercises may help you prevent falls.

How? The drills used in balance training strengthen muscles that keep you stable and upright, particularly in your legs and core. And while balance training may help you avoid fall-related injury, that's not all it does.

One study showed that four months of a high-intensity, balance-focused functional exercise program helped seniors with non-Alzheimer's dementia continue activities of daily living longer. That's compared to a control group that participated in seated activities.

Balancing trains your brain. Researchers also studied balance training in healthy people age 18 to 65 over a 12-week period. Twice a week, participants worked through eight five-minute exercises.

The result? Their memory improved, and so did their spatial thinking — the mental skill you need to pack a box or learn your way around a new building. Researchers think balance training stimulates your sensory system which may encourage changes in parts of your brain involved in memory and spatial tasks.

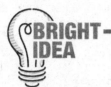

BRIGHT IDEA

Get your sea legs back with these exercises

On March 5, 2020, Nik Wallenda became the first person to walk a tightrope across an active volcano — and it was broadcast live on television. Now that's putting your balance training to the test. Fortunately you don't need the drama of a volcano to show off your skills. These simple exercises will have your balancing act ready in no time.

Heel to toe. Walk a straight line by placing the heel of one foot directly in front of the toes of your other foot. Hold your arms out to your sides for balance. After 10 steps, turn around and go back to your starting point the same way. Repeat this exercise 10 times.

Body circles. Stand with your feet shoulder-width apart. While you keep your body straight and your feet flat, slowly sway in a circle, rotating clockwise for 30 to 60 seconds. Pause, then repeat the exercise in the opposite direction.

Single-leg stand. With your feet together and your arms to your sides, lift one leg as high as you can. Balance on one foot for about 10 seconds. You may want to support your lifted leg with both hands just under the knee, or hold on to a chair, counter, or wall as a prop. Repeat with the other leg. Do five repetitions.

Back leg raises. Stand behind a chair and hold for support. Lift your right leg straight back and hold the position for about two seconds without bending your knees. Try not to lean forward. Return your leg to the original position, then repeat the exercise on the other leg. Do 15 repetitions.

Top tips to break your fall risk

Remember spinning around as a child, purposely making yourself dizzy till you tumbled to the floor? It was a lot of fun years ago, but the thought of it now might make you green around the gills. Maybe that's nature's way of telling you that feeling lightheaded and wobbly is no laughing matter once you've passed a certain age.

In fact, toppling over after a dizzy spell can be downright scary. And many seniors, even if they don't get hurt, become afraid it will happen again. So they become less active, which increases their risk of taking a spill in the future. How can you avoid the fear of the fall? The answer's almost too good to be true.

> Ever feel woozy — like you can't shake the feeling you're moving — after watching an action movie? You might be experiencing visually induced motion sickness, a sensory mismatch that happens when you see movement but can't feel it. Don't let it throw you off balance. Give your eyes frequent breaks from visual stimuli, and be careful when standing.

Simple ways to prevent falls and conquer dizzy spells — no pills required. Remove clutter from your floors and toss out slippery throw rugs. You'll avoid tumbles, and as a bonus, your house will stay neat as a pin. And don't forget, exercise in your freshly tidied house will improve lower body strength and help you with walking and balance.

As for dizziness — which affects 30% of people 60 and older — here's what to do. If you feel woozy, lie down on a sofa or bed to encourage blood flow to your brain. After a few minutes, sit up gradually. Stay sitting for a few more minutes before slowly rising to your feet.

Stop, drop, and roll like a pro. Despite your best efforts, you may still find yourself tilt to the point of tipping over. More than 1 in 4 Americans 65 and older takes a tumble each year, and about 20% of those falls lead to a fracture or worse. Instead of becoming a fall statistic, channel your inner stunt person and practice these four techniques to help you fall more safely and avoid a life-altering injury.

Step 1. Loosen up for a softer landing.

Step 2. Protect your head.

Step 3. Land on the meaty parts of your body.

Step 4. Keep rolling to lessen injury.

Don't confuse this common condition with dementia

Annie noticed her mom wasn't as steady on her feet as she used to be. Even more concerning, her mom was forgetting birthdays and other things she had always been keen to remember. When she also developed incontinence, Annie couldn't shake the nagging question — was it dementia? After some investigation, thankfully it wasn't.

A condition called normal pressure hydrocephalus can mimic those symptoms. In adults over age 50, fluid may build up inside the skull over time instead of being reabsorbed by the body as it should. That puts pressure on the brain, which is when you start to notice these kinds of worrisome changes.

- difficulty walking, or a shuffling gait
- slower thinking, delayed responses
- poor memory

Normal pressure hydrocephalus can be hard to diagnose because it so closely resembles other conditions. Fortunately it's usually treatable through surgery.

Berries

Build up your brain with berried treasure

Brilliant berries. Raspberries, blackberries, cranberries, and the luscious list goes on. Berries contain pigments called anthocyanins that create the rainbow of colors you love — and the health benefits you crave. Jam-packed with an alphabet of nutrients like vitamins C, A, and K, along with fiber and minerals, these juicy little gems are great for your heart, bones, and skin — well, just about all of you.

But if you're looking for an especially brain-healthy berry, you've got to go for the blue.

Thanks for the memories, blueberries. Can you believe it? This little berry gives your brain the nutrients it needs for a better memory.

> Folklore says bilberries — a cousin of blueberries — improve your eyesight. The story goes that British pilots in World War II filled up on bilberry jam to sharpen their night vision. Some say that was just a rumor cooked up to keep the Germans from discovering new radar equipment on British planes. Still, bilberries have healthy antioxidants that hunt down disease-promoting free radicals.

In a study of more than 200 volunteers, age 60 to 70, folks were given either a daily dose of blueberry-grape extract or a placebo. After six months, the researchers concluded that the extract improved age-related losses in the episodic memories — the memory of everyday events — of the seniors with the most cognitive decline.

And more studies done with older adults, including those with mild cognitive impairment (MCI), suggest that blueberries benefit executive function — the skills you need to pay attention, set goals, and remember instructions, for example — and psychomotor function, which lets you control your movements. MCI is the stage between the normal cognitive decline associated with aging and the more serious decline of dementia.

Blueberries fine-tune your brain. Want to improve your cognitive abilities? Treat yourself to a bowl of blueberries every day. In one study, a small group of folks between the ages of 60 and 75 ate either freeze-dried blueberries — equal to 1 cup of fresh berries — or a placebo daily over 90 days. At the end of the study, the seniors who ate the freeze-dried blueberries had fewer errors on verbal memory and task-switching tests compared with the control group.

Another study showed that folks who ate a diet with a similar amount of freeze-dried blueberries felt their cognition had improved, especially as it related to activities of everyday life, like eating, bathing, and walking.

Cherry, banana, watermelon. One of these fruits is not a berry. Can you guess which one? If you guessed watermelon or banana, you'd be wrong. They're berries. Surely a cherry is a berry? Nope. According to folks-in-the-know, a berry must have more than one seed. Other surprise berries include eggplants and kiwis.

Outsmart Alzheimer's disease (AD). Remember, blueberries are packed with anthocyanins, powerful antioxidants that can stave off diseases of aging, like Alzheimer's — the most common form of dementia.

In one small study, seniors age 68 and older with MCI were given either freeze-dried blueberry powder — equal to a cup of berries — or a placebo powder once a day for 16 weeks. At the end of the study, the researchers found that the seniors who ate the blueberry powder experienced improvements in their brain function and cognition compared with the placebo group.

Scientists hope anthocyanins, like those found in blueberries, may turn out to be an inexpensive way to ward off age-related diseases that affect the brain, including AD.

Protect yourself from Parkinson's disease (PD). Blueberries to the rescue — again. A 20-year study of the dietary habits of 130,000 adults found that men who ate the most flavonoid-rich foods — including blueberries — were 40% less likely to develop PD than men who ate the least. Oddly enough, no similar link was found for total flavonoid intake in women.

In PD, dopaninergic neurons — the main source of dopamine — die off. Dopamine is a chemical that relays signals between nerve cells that control movement. When dopaninergic neurons die off, symptoms of PD like slowness, stiffness, and balance problems happen. Flavonoids in berries may protect against the oxidative stress that damages dopamine neurons.

Don't let your brain deteriorate when you can so easily power it up with flavonoid-rich fruits like blueberries.

A little blue juice keeps you in the pink

You already know that the good-for-you anthocyanins jammed into blueberries keep your brain sharp. Here's another way to amp up those anthocynanins — juice 'em. One study showed just 2 cups of blueberry juice every day improved learning and word list recall. Wonder what else this purply-blue delight can do for you? Here are three good reasons you should drink this every day.

Lower blood pressure with blueberry juice. High blood pressure is the biggest risk factor for heart disease. And it can lead to heart attack, stroke, kidney damage, memory loss, and vision loss. But don't worry. Blueberries are here to keep your numbers where they need to be.

A small study comparing blueberry juice to control drinks found that participants who drank blueberry juice daily for one month saw, on average, a 5-point reduction in blood pressure. The researchers say similar results are commonly seen in folks taking blood pressure meds.

They also found that the anthocyanins in blueberries improved endothelial function. Endothelial cells play a key role in regulating blood pressure, and blueberries' anthocyanins give the cells the healthy boost they need.

Blueberries provide a feast for your eyes. With aging comes a breakdown of the retinal pigment epithelial (RPE) cells in your eyes — a common cause of macular degeneration. But a study on stressed RPE cells in a petri dish found that those bathed in blueberry anthocyanins were exposed to fewer free radicals — rogue molecules that damage cells — and had a lower amount of aged cells.

And a separate study of more than 35,000 women over the age of 45 suggests that eating blueberries reduces the risk of age-related macular degeneration. Researchers say more work needs to be done in this area, but they're betting the anthocyanins in blueberries may help you see through healthier eyes.

Maintain a healthy weight with blueberries. Lots of seniors struggle to keep their weight in check. But too much weight gain raises your risk of conditions linked to dementia, including heart disease. Fortunately, blueberries may help keep you slim and trim.

A 24-year study of more than 133,000 adults suggests that the more blueberries you eat, the less weight you gain as you age. And separate research on some 2,700 healthy female twins found that the twin who ate more blueberries had lower fat mass and less belly fat. And you know why? You can probably guess. Yep, the anthocyanins.

Color your table with nutritious berries

Berries are bright and beautiful, and as fresh and delicious as a bowl of summer sunshine. But what's all this stuff about nutrition? From blackberries to raspberries, here's the scoop on the vitamins and minerals found in berries, and how they can help you stay healthy.

Nutrient	Sources	Health benefits
Fiber	blackberries, boysenberries, cranberries, elderberries, loganberries, raspberries	Fiber helps with weight control. Berries are a good source of soluble fiber, the kind that slows the movement of food through your digestive tract and makes you feel full for longer periods.
Vitamin C	blackberries, blueberries, elderberries, gooseberries, mulberries, raspberries	Vitamin C may help protect you from chronic conditions like heart disease. It boosts your immune system, and studies suggest it protects your memory and thinking.
Manganese	blackberries, blueberries, boysenberries, grapes, loganberries, raspberries	Manganese is important for bone development and may protect you from osteoporosis. It boosts your immune system and may help manage blood sugar levels.
Vitamin K	blackberries, blueberries, boysenberries, grapes, mulberries, raspberries	You need vitamin K for blood clotting and wound healing. And vitamin K has been linked to good bone health.
Iron	blackberries, blueberries, boysenberries, elderberries, loganberries, raspberries	Iron is an important part of hemoglobin, the component of red blood cells that carries oxygen to your cells. You can boost your body's ability to absorb iron by eating foods that are high in vitamin C.
Potassium	blackberries, elderberries, gooseberries, grapes, mulberries, raspberries	The potassium in berries may help keep your blood pressure in check.
Folate	blackberries, blueberries, boysenberries, elderberries, loganberries, raspberries	The folate found in berries may help protect your heart. And folate deficiency has been linked to depression.

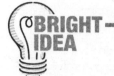

Keep your berries straight-from-the-farm fresh

A little berry humor for you. What do you call a sad raspberry? A "blue" berry, of course. Terrible joke, isn't it? But even more terrible is bringing home beautiful berries and watching them go bad because they weren't washed and stored properly. Follow the tips below to keep your berries as fresh and sweet as the day they were picked.

- When choosing your berries, look for those that are tender, juicy, and brightly colored. Beware of containers that are damp or stained. Select berries that pull away easily from their stems.

- As soon as you get them home, put them in the fridge for about an hour. They'll firm up a little which makes them easier to rinse.

- Just before you're ready to use them, place your berries in a colander and rinse them under gently running water. No need to soak. To make your berries last longer try adding some apple cider vinegar to the wash. Fill a bowl with 3 cups of water and add 1 cup of apple cider vinegar. Pour in your unwashed berries and stir them with your hands. Repeat the process with plain water so you don't end up with vinegar-flavored berries.

- After they're washed, leave them in the colander. Place the colander inside a large bowl to allow air to circulate around the berries and dry them. And skip the crisper. Berry buffs believe your fruit will go bad more quickly because the air in the crisper has higher humidity and doesn't circulate as much as in the rest of the fridge.

Brain training

Put your brain on a powerlifting plan

The strongest men in the world can lift 900-pound weights straight off the ground. Their stunning brute strength might be helpful on occasion, but wouldn't you rather have an agile brain? You already know you can improve your physical condition with the right kind of exercise. But you can also improve your memory and thinking skills with brain training — regular, repeated mental tasks that get progressively more challenging.

Choose mind over memory exercises for lasting effects. Sometimes you just need to remember which groceries to buy later in the day. For tasks like that, memorization tricks can help you jog specific memories. But when you want to improve mental skills like being able to think faster or tune up your laser-like focus on a problem, you'll need something a little more rigorous. Enter brain training.

- Researchers at the University of Texas at Dallas studied the effects of a program called Strategic Memory Advanced Reasoning Training (SMART) over 12 weeks. They reported in *Neurobiology of Aging* that this cognitive training helped seniors' brains work more efficiently on tasks — much like younger brains.

- A separate study looked at the effects of an eight-week brain training program on older adults with mild cognitive impairment. After participating in the training sessions for two hours each week, the seniors increased their memory scores by 35%

to 40%. They maintained those scores during the six-month follow-up. Plus they reported using the strategies they learned from the program in their daily lives.

Build your own brain training program. The key to giving your brain the best workout is to make sure you include a variety of activities that target multiple skills and stimulate your whole brain.

- Focus your attention without distractions twice a day at least 30 minutes at a time. Don't try to multitask.

- Pick up a new skill like digital photography or blogging. Complex tasks like these engage your brain in specific functions like problem-solving and creative thinking. Make sure the activity is both different and hard enough to pose a challenge for you.

> Contrary to what anyone might tell you, multitasking is not a superpower. Forcing your brain to toggle between tasks kills your attention span and the quality of your work. And if you're multitasking and trying to learn something new, you may find it more difficult to commit information to memory.

- Change up your routine for a familiar task like how you put your dishes away.

- Explain a complicated task like cooking your favorite meal as if you were telling a child how to do it. Your brain has to work hard to make that information easy to understand.

- After learning new information — say, from watching an educational Ted Talk video online — take a few moments to figure out the big idea being discussed. Ask yourself how you could relate it to your daily life. For more challenge, put your brain to work explaining what you have learned to someone else. That helps you uncover gaps in your understanding.

- Think long term. Your retirement account wasn't funded in one day. Neither will your brain change overnight. Practice will ultimately help you see improvements in targeted brain functions.

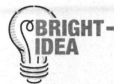

Make your noggin nimbler with neurobics

You've probably noticed fitness centers in your hometown. Wouldn't it be great if you could drop your brain off at one for a little treadmill work every day to improve its performance? Fortunately, you can help keep your brain fit with neurobic exercises, mental fitness workouts for your brain cells, or neurons.

As a type of brain training, the goal of these exercises is to work your brain in unexpected ways. Shake up your routines, and use your environment to challenge yourself. Some experts say the more you engage your senses with activities like these, the better your brain's fitness and flexibility.

- Visit a new place. Maybe it's a different coffee shop, a new state. Or eat lunch somewhere different like the great outdoors.

- Use your television remote control or computer mouse with your nondominant hand.

- Take a different path to your favorite shopping place. Notice the signs and landmarks along the way as if you wanted to tell someone else how to take that route. Even natural features like the smell of evergreens activate pathways in your brain.

- Test your touch. Drop random coins in your pocket. Try to name each coin as you fish it out based only on its surface features. Make it more challenging by adding international coins to the mix. If you're short on change, try finding your favorite shirt using only your sense of touch.

- Pull out your spice rack and identify your herbs and spices by smell.

Broccoli

Broccoli beats back Alzheimer's and ups your metabolism

Looking for the perfect veggie side dish? You can find this tree-shaped treat in nearly every grocery store. Even better, this one amazing vegetable — broccoli — may fight off Alzheimer's disease (AD) and slow the aging process. No wonder it's often called the crown jewel of nutrition.

Sulforaphane prevents Alzheimer's plaque. The buildup and clumping of the protein beta-amyloid in your brain can have devastating effects — like contributing to the development of AD. But a plaque-busting compound in broccoli called sulforaphane may help prevent this disease.

Sulforaphane energizes your immune system and has antioxidant and anti-inflammatory properties. Testing on mice suggests it can also stop the formation of beta-amyloid. Researchers say sulforaphane has the potential to lower beta-amyloid buildup in people with AD, too. This may be because sulforaphane increases levels of a protein — dubbed CHIP, for short — that helps prevent the accumulation of beta-amyloid in the brain.

Save your sniffer from broccoli's unappetizing odor with a little vinegar. Pour undiluted white vinegar into a bowl, and set it near the broccoli as it cooks to counteract the smell. Turn on the exhaust fan over your stove and keep your cooking time to a minimum.

Boost your metabolism to slow down aging. Your cells' ability to produce energy declines as you get older. This loss of efficiency in your body's energy supply may be a key player in aging. That's why researchers think NAD — a coenzyme essential to energy production — may reduce some of the typical signs of aging.

But a mouse study by the Washington University School of Medicine showed that taking NAD directly doesn't work. That's where an NAD-boosting compound called NMN comes in. Researchers found that NMN, when given to mice in their drinking water, converts to NAD in the body. But only older mice saw improvements in age-related health issues that can affect the brain like poor vision, insulin sensitivity, and weight gain.

"NMN supplementation has no effect in the young mice because they are still making plenty of their own NMN," says co-senior author of the study Jun Yoshino, M.D., Ph.D. "We suspect that the increase in inflammation that happens with aging reduces the body's ability to make NMN and, by extension, NAD."

Further studies are needed to see if similar benefits translate to humans. But you can get plenty of NMN in broccoli. Other great sources include cabbage, cucumber, edamame, and avocado.

Sprout's honor: Feast your way to better health

Bite-sized candy bars are sweet little treats, but you'll get mega health benefits in more natural fun-sized snacks. Baby carrots and palm-sized clementines are tasty choices. But if you want to pack a punch against diabetes, choose lesser-known broccoli sprouts.

Diabetes is bad news for your memory. It damages your blood vessels and hampers oxygen flow to your brain. But broccoli sprouts help you avoid blood sugar spikes that, over time, harm brain cells.

The compound helping out is called sulforaphane. And these three-day-old broccoli plants provide even more of it than mature broccoli. So what does sulforaphane do?

Broccoli sprouts lower blood sugar levels. If you have type 2 diabetes, sulforaphane may be just what you need to improve fasting glucose levels — your blood sugar after fasting overnight — and decrease glycated hemoglobin (HbA1c) levels. Doctors measure HbA1c to determine your average blood sugar over several weeks or months.

In a study published by *Science Translational Medicine*, 97 participants with type 2 diabetes received either a daily dose of concentrated broccoli sprout extract or a placebo. After three months, the researchers found improved fasting glucose levels among the extract takers with "dysregulated" diabetes — those who had high glucose levels at the start of the study. In addition, obese volunteers with high starting glucose levels saw significant drops in their HbA1c levels.

The researchers say sulforaphane improves glucose levels by suppressing liver enzymes involved in its production.

> Human brains have gotten significantly smaller over the last 10,000 to 20,000 years. How much has been lost? A chunk about the size of a tennis ball. You can't do anything about that, but you can make smarter food choices to give your brain the nourishment it needs. The ball is in your court.

Help your heart with a supplement. As if that's not enough, research suggests that broccoli sprouts can also improve your cholesterol levels. A study published in the journal *Diabetes Research and Clinical Practice* analyzed people with type 2 diabetes who took a broccoli sprout powder supplement daily for four weeks. The researchers saw significant decreases in their serum triglycerides — a type of fat in the blood — as well as their ratios of oxidized LDL to LDL cholesterol.

High levels of triglycerides and oxidized LDL — "bad" cholesterol that becomes even more dangerous after chemical interactions with free radicals — are both linked to an increased risk of stroke, heart attack, and heart disease. That may be why sprouts are a boon for your ticker.

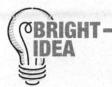

Make the most of your meal with these tips

Sulforaphane — that beneficial plant compound found in cruciferous vegetables like broccoli, cabbage, cauliflower, and kale — offers a slew of benefits, from your head to your heart. But the amount you get from your food depends on how you prepare it. Here's how to get the most from your meals.

Unlike some other nutrients, sulforaphane isn't readily available in vegetables — it has to be made. When you chomp into a piece of broccoli, for example, the plant compound glucoraphanin converts into sulforaphane. Other damage to a broccoli stalk — like cutting and chopping — sparks this change, too.

Keep your veggies raw to be rewarded with the highest levels of this healthy compound. Crudités not your thing? Although cooking can decrease the sulforaphane in your broccoli, you can limit the loss with these tricks.

- Lightly steam for one to three minutes.

- Skip the microwave — the high temperature can destroy glucoraphanin before it has a chance to convert.

- Reduce the amount of water you use if boiling. The health benefits can get lost in the cooking water.

- Minimize cook time. The longer you leave your broccoli boiling, the more glucoraphanin you lose.

If you have some extra prep time on your hands, chop up your broccoli before stir-frying. Let the pieces sit for 90 minutes. Why? Research suggests the wait time allows sulforaphane to develop.

Get even more of this sulfur-rich compound by sprinkling mustard seeds or mustard powder on your broccoli. The spice boosts the availability of sulforaphane, particularly in cooked vegetables.

Caffeine

Memory maximizer: A natural way to chase away forgetfulness

Did you know bees get a buzz when they drink from flowers with caffeinated nectar? Caffeine appears to support long-term memory in your honey-making friends, and it may boost your brainpower, too.

Whether you get it from a plant, medicine, food, or drink, caffeine is a fast-acting stimulant that ramps up your energy level. Ordinarily, a chemical in your body called adenosine links up with areas on cells called adenosine receptors. This binding slows nerve cell activity and causes you to wind down or feel sleepy. But caffeine blocks the effect of adenosine, so you feel perked up and attentive instead.

This action helps your brain in two powerful ways.

Caffeine keeps dementia at bay.

In the 10-year Women's Health Initiative Memory Study of 6,467 women age 65 and older, those who said they drank more than 261 milligrams (mg) of caffeine a day — what you would get from drinking up to 3 cups of coffee or 6 cups of black tea — were 36% less likely to develop cognitive impairment or dementia than women who consumed a low amount of caffeine.

Wish you could be a little quicker on the uptake? Researchers reported at an annual Cognitive Neuroscience Society meeting that just one caffeinated drink improved reaction time and accuracy on attention tests for people 55 and older — even after being off caffeine for a solid week.

Experts continue to study caffeine's effects on the brain. But many point to its ability to block adenosine receptors, which may not function as well as you get older and could be partially responsible for age-related changes in cognition.

Need to perk up your memory? Caffeine does the trick. Ever notice little changes like when a neighbor plants new flowers in front of her house? If so, you're using your memory to distinguish between similar situations, something called pattern separation. That means you pick up on slight differences in how something appears now compared with the last time you saw it.

Researchers at Johns Hopkins University discovered caffeine can help this process. They asked 160 adults who didn't usually eat or drink caffeine to study various pictures. Five minutes later, the volunteers took either a pill containing 200 mg of caffeine — about the same amount as in 2 small cups of coffee — or a placebo.

The participants came back 24 hours later — the amount of time it would take for the caffeine to leave their system — and researchers showed them a set of pictures again. This time, some of the pictures were new, others were the same, and the rest had small differences from the ones they saw the day before.

The big difference between the caffeine and placebo groups? The caffeine group was significantly better at correctly identifying similar photos instead of mistakenly citing them as the same. The researchers think the results may be caused by caffeine's ability to prevent adenosine from blocking the release of a memory-assisting chemical called norepinephrine.

Manage a migraine and beat the blues

People who suffer from migraine are five times more likely to develop depression. Challenging as both conditions can be, help could be waiting in your favorite caffeinated food and drink.

Caffeine heads off headache pain. Complain of a headache to an Italian grandmother and she might strap potato slices to your forehead with strict instructions to rest for 30 minutes. But it might be easier to pick up a caffeinated drink and an over-the-counter (OTC) pain killer.

When it comes to headaches, research suggests caffeine makes a good side kick to OTC pain relievers like acetaminophen and nonsteroidal anti-inflammatory drugs (NSAIDs) like aspirin and ibuprofen. Results of a study reported in *The Journal of Headache and Pain* found that migraine sufferers who took a combo of 500 milligrams (mg) of acetaminophen, 500 mg of aspirin, and 130 mg of caffeine had less pain and fewer migraine-related symptoms than those who took a placebo.

Caffeine may head migraine misery off at the pass, but a new study in *The American Journal of Medicine* cautions migraine sufferers to limit themselves to two caffeinated drinks a day. Researchers say you increase your odds of triggering a migraine within 24 hours if you go over that amount.

Migraines differ from tension headaches because they often come with nausea, vomiting, and increased sensitivity to light, smell, and sound. A separate study on people with tension headaches found that volunteers who took 400 mg of ibuprofen and 200 mg of caffeine felt greater pain relief than control groups that took ibuprofen alone, caffeine alone, or a placebo. No wonder pain relievers often have caffeine as an ingredient.

Caffeine lifts you up when you're down. Legend has it that an Ethiopian shepherd discovered coffee after he found his goats bouncing with energy after eating the berries. Wouldn't it be great to have that enthusiasm to overcome the blues? Maybe you can.

Caffeine doesn't just improve your mood. A review of multiple studies suggests it may help prevent mild to moderate depression. Researchers found that people who took between 68 mg and 509 mg of caffeine a day were less likely to become depressed. Just 2 cups of black tea, for example, contain nearly 100 mg.

How might caffeine work on depression? Researchers believe caffeine enhances the effectiveness of the "feel-good" chemical dopamine in the front part of your brain. That's where motivation, decision making, and sense of reward all take place.

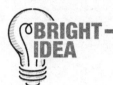

BRIGHT IDEA

Can't sleep? Look out for hidden sources of caffeine

Experts suggest you keep your daily tally of caffeine at 400 milligrams (mg) or less. If you're counting, you probably included your pain relievers. But did you know dietary supplements and weight loss pills can pack a caffeine punch of as much as 1,200 mg? That's the same amount of caffeine you'd get from 12 cups of coffee.

Since food manufacturers don't have to list caffeine on their product labels, it's tricky to know how much you're really getting. Before you finish your caffeine calculations, don't forget to include these less obvious sources of caffeine in your diet.

Food	Serving size	Caffeine (mg)
energy drink	8.3 ounces	75
chocolate cake mix	1 package	57.6
noncola soda	12 ounces	53.2
chocolate candy bar	1 bar	27.1
chocolate-flavored carbonated drink	12 ounces	7.4
chocolate frozen yogurt	1 cup	5.2
cocoa, hot	1 envelope	5
chocolate milk	1 cup	2.5
decaf coffee	8 ounces	2.4
decaf tea	8 ounces	2.4
protein bar	1 bar	2.4
chocolate pudding	4 ounces	2.2
chocolate ice cream	1/2 cup	2

Carbohydrates

Brain bonus — 3 fast facts about the benefits of carbs

This food type may get a bad rap from weight loss gurus, but carbohydrates are essential to keep you moving. Carbs fuel your brain and nervous system, and they keep your digestive system regular, too.

Experts recommend you get your fill of this body booster by choosing a type called complex carbohydrates. These carbs have three or more sugar molecules joined together in long, complex structures. That design means your body puts in more work to break them down than simple carbs, which are more easily digested and absorbed, often leading to swinging blood sugar levels and weight gain.

The best complex carbs are those that have not been refined, meaning nutrients like fiber haven't been stripped out during processing. Where refined foods like cookies and bagels can contribute to weight gain and high blood sugar, whole and minimally processed foods do the opposite.

So pop a bowl of popcorn — it's a whole grain, making it a high-quality source of carbs — and sit back and learn how eating complex carbohydrates can be a boon for your brain health.

Get an energy boost with carbs. For an easy way to fuel your body, carbs are a must-eat. They break down into the sugar glucose, which is used by tissues and cells throughout your body. When you don't get enough carbs, your body may get energy by breaking down proteins into glucose. That's bad news because you need those proteins to build your muscles.

Call it picky, but your brain needs carbs for energy. That makes them essential to your nervous system. If you don't have enough glucose in your body, you may feel dizzy and weak. But complex carbs can keep your energy at an even keel.

Carbs are good for your gut. Fiber is a type of carbohydrate your gut can't digest. It slows food breakdown and keeps you regular by helping move waste out.

Hey big spender! Your brain uses up to 25% of your energy budget — more than any other organ in your body. And when it comes to your blood glucose, your thinking cap uses as much as 60% of what's available. Plus it requires more glucose when it's working extra hard during challenging mental tasks.

Plus when your gut bacteria break down undigested complex carbs, they create helpful fatty acids that improve your gut health. But the benefits don't stop there. Experts say these fatty acids may also impact your mood and memory.

Improve your sleep with this late-night snack. Ever feel sleepy straight after eating a big meal? You can blame the nap-inducing amino acid tryptophan. Carbs make it easier for your brain to absorb tryptophan, so a loaded plate may sweep you off to sweet dreams faster than you expect. But that's just what your brain needs. Not getting enough sleep can hurt your memory and ability to pay attention.

Pair your carbs with a protein for an even better evening snack. Proteins are the building block of tryptophan, so peanut butter on toast could be your perfect send-off to dreamland.

How carbs help you get a handle on your weight and blood sugar

Carbs go above and beyond to keep you healthy. They spread benefits throughout your body by fighting two big conditions that take a blow to your brain health.

Carbs weigh in on shedding pounds. Studies have shown time and again that eating more carbs is associated with less risk of being overweight. Just make sure you eat the right kind, say researchers in a recent large study. The trial, known as the Diabetes Prevention Program, studied nearly 3,000 people with a high risk of diabetes. Their weight loss after one year was related to eating more carbs, specifically fiber, and less fat.

Add more fiber into your diet with an extra serving of vegetables every day. The crunchy cruciferous kind — think broccoli, cabbage, and cauliflower — are a great option. Eating more fruit and high-fiber, low-fat grains can improve weight loss, too. Because they turn down the dial on digestion speed, you feel full longer and absorb sugars more slowly.

These changes are ideal for achieving your weight loss and maintenance goals in the long run, which is great for your brain because obesity raises your risk of developing conditions linked to dementia.

Keep your blood sugar under control with carbs. The authors of the previously mentioned weight loss study, published in *The Journal of Nutrition*, emphasize that losing weight may protect high-risk individuals from getting diabetes. But weight loss isn't the only way carbs help your fight against diabetes. They also get to the heart of your problem — your blood sugar.

Resistant starch is a type of carb that isn't digested in the small intestine. That's why it's also considered a fiber. Compared to digestible carbs, resistant starch lowers your glycemic response, or the effect food has on your blood sugar. That means it helps even out your blood sugar levels, fighting off unwanted spikes or crashes.

And the reason may be because it increases the production of certain fatty acids in your gut that influence insulin sensitivity. That's good news for your noggin since spikes in blood sugar damage brain cells. Get your fill naturally from bananas, potatoes, grains, and legumes.

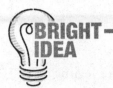 **BRIGHT IDEA**

All fab, no fad:
The best way to get carbs

Fad diets may have you convinced that cutting all carbs is the key to good health. But with your body so reliant on this food group, the real health trick is to find carbs that are fab — fabulous, that is.

Empty calories, also called empty carbs, are the real enemy. Processing has stripped them of valuable nutrients like vitamins and fiber. So instead of skipping all carbs, just ditch the refined ones.

Some refined foods are obvious. White bread, white rice, and pastries, which are all packed with refined grains, don't try and trick you into thinking they're healthy. Same with foods high in refined sugar like cakes, condiments, and soda.

But don't fall for the ruse of wheat or multigrain bread. These names are marketing ploys — they don't mean the loaf is made from unprocessed whole grains like many people assume. Instead, scan the label for "100% whole wheat" or "100% whole grain" to ensure you're buying a whole food.

And that's not all. Instant oatmeal is only masquerading as the perfect breakfast. All the added sugars are refined carbs you don't need. Opt for rolled or steel-cut oats, and skip or add a smidge of sugar yourself.

Your body digests highly processed carbs like these too quickly to give you lasting energy. They may even spike your blood sugar and bring on "brain fog." When that happens you may feel like it's harder to focus or remember things. But cutting out those carbs can clear your mind. Fill their place with vitamin- and mineral-packed complex carbs like spinach, whole barley, grapefruit, buckwheat, and apples.

Lift your mood and sharpen your mind guilt-free

You may find yourself sneaking extra snacks when you're feeling down. But with a shift in the glycemic load of your diet, you may not feel down to start with.

Glycemic load (GL) gauges how a carb, and how much of it you eat, affects your blood sugar level. And the concentration of glucose running through your veins influences your brain health, from mood to memory.

Delicious foods kick the blues. In a study of 82 adults, researchers found a link between depression and diet. Those with a high-glycemic load diet experienced more symptoms of depression than those with a low-GL diet. This was especially noticeable in people who were overweight but otherwise healthy.

And shifting to low-GL foods may make your taste buds happy, too. In the study, folks switched high-GL foods such as plain white bagels and instant mashed potatoes for tasty low-GL foods like whole-grain pumpernickel bread and barley pilaf. Yum.

The right meal plan keeps you sharp as a tack. Watching your GL can also help your thinking skills, says a study published in *Clinical Nutrition* that followed almost 200 cognitively healthy seniors.

Researchers didn't find a link between GL and cognition for folks who had well-regulated glucose. But for people with poorly regulated glucose levels, a diet with a low glycemic load was linked to better cognitive function — mental abilities that involve learning, problem-solving, and processing and storing information.

Ready to help your brain and make a change? Lowering your glycemic load may be as simple as a few diet swaps. Trade out starchy foods like potatoes and white rice and add in whole grains and nonstarchy veggies. Nuts and legumes are great additions, too.

Watch out for ketogenic 'wonder' diet

Cutting down on carbohydrates is a core tenet of the keto-genic diet, or keto. But is dropping carbs from your meal plan right for you? Time to straighten out the truth.

Where you may normally get half of your energy from carbs, keto drops that to less than one-tenth. Instead, fat becomes your prime fuel source, and its breakdown — called ketosis — creates molecules known as ketone bodies. These chemicals may be behind the brain benefits of the keto diet. That's according to early research that suggests the keto may help reduce symptoms of Parkinson's and Alzheimer's disease.

But before you go all in on the keto diet, know that it has risks, too — especially for the older set. It may lower your appetite and nutrient intake, putting you at risk for malnutrition. Plus it's been linked to nausea, constipation, and dehydration. More research is needed before researchers can back this low-carb craze.

Chamomile

Feeling anxious? Try this tonic in a teapot

With a tummy packed full of fresh veggies, a frightened Peter Rabbit barely escaped Mr. McGregor's garden. And by the time he'd hopped all the way home, he had an awful stomachache caused by his terrifying encounter with the angry gardener — and too many French beans. Mrs. Rabbit's cure? A tablespoon of chamomile tea to calm his nerves.

Chamomile tea may seem a bit old-fashioned — after all, the Egyptians wrote about chugging the tasty tea way back in 1550 B.C. But it's kept up with the times when it comes to soothing anxiety and helping depression. Chamomile is a calming, naturally caffeine-free tea that also acts as an anti-inflammatory, an ulcer-fighter, an antioxidant, and an antimicrobial. Good choice, Mrs. Rabbit.

Ease anxiety with a soothing cup. Symptoms of generalized anxiety disorder (GAD) include excessive worry, restlessness, fatigue, irritability, muscle tension, and sleep problems.

In a study of 57 people with mild to moderate GAD, 28 were given a daily capsule containing 220 milligrams of chamomile while the remaining 29 were given a placebo. Doses increased to two capsules a day during the second week, and up to five capsules a day in the following weeks. By the end of the eight-week study, the people taking chamomile showed significant improvements on tests that measure anxiety.

Depression takes a dive. As a follow-up to this study, researchers looked at the effects of chamomile on depression. They saw a greater reduction in symptoms of depression in the people taking chamomile than those taking a placebo. The researchers concluded that flavonoids in chamomile may have antidepressant as well as anti-anxiety properties.

Make your own chamomile tea. You can make delicious chamomile tea faster than Peter Rabbit ran through the garden. Start with 3 to 4 tablespoons of dried chamomile — you can find it at a farmers market or online — and add hot water. Steep for up to 10 minutes. If you prefer fresh chamomile, let it steep for about three minutes. Of course, if you're not a tea drinker, you can always get chamomile in supplement form instead.

Tea for 2: Chamomile controls blood sugar and eases inflammation

Steamed over your high blood sugar? Rheumatoid arthritis pain brewing? Better health is in the bag. The tea bag, that is. A cuppa chamomile may be just the natural remedy you need to wash away your symptoms.

> Chamomile does it all. It can be used as a tea, a lotion, capsules, or drops. And it's simply blooming with health benefits. Use it to treat cuts and scrapes, rashes, burns — even dark circles under your eyes. It's good for toothaches and migraines, too.

Cozy up to chamomile for better blood sugar. High blood sugar can damage the small blood vessels and nerves in your brain. And that can lead to vascular cognitive impairment or vascular dementia. But researchers think chamomile tea after every meal may help improve your blood sugar control.

The study included 64 adults with type 2 diabetes who were divided into two groups. Both groups kept their usual diet, but the first one drank chamomile tea — one 3-gram bag steeped in a little more than 1/2 cup of water for 10 minutes — three times a day for eight weeks. The control group drank only warm water after each meal. By the end of the study, the A1C — average blood sugar — of the chamomile drinkers dropped 5% compared with an increase of almost 1% in the control group.

Researchers — and tea drinkers — are encouraged by these results, but further testing is needed.

Chamomile "leaves" inflammation behind. If you suffer from rheumatoid arthritis (RA), you may understand what it feels like to be in a brain fog. The inflammation caused by this disease can affect parts of the brain that help you make decisions, consolidate new memories, and retrieve information from your long-term memory.

But RA also attacks the lining of your joints. You may have tender, swollen joints in your fingers and toes. And as the disease progresses, symptoms can move to your wrists, knees, elbows, and ankles. Fortunately, researchers think chamomile tea may help.

> Do you get allergy symptoms like watery eyes or sinus pressure during ragweed season? If so, avoid chamomile. Ragweed and chamomile are kissin' cousins that can trigger serious allergic reactions, including a swollen throat, rapid pulse, and hives. Other plants to avoid? Daisy, chrysanthemum, and marigold can spark the same alarming response.

A group of women with RA between the ages of 20 and 65 participated in a study about the effects of this soothing drink. They were divided into two groups. One was given a little more than 1/2 cup of chamomile tea after lunch and dinner each day for six weeks. The other was given wheat bran tea that had the same color and herbal fragrance as the chamomile tea. At the end of the study, the chamomile drinkers had fewer tender joints and their ESR — a measure of inflammation in the body — was lower.

So what's in this little cup of tea that can make such a big difference for RA sufferers? Researchers think it may be a flavonoid called apigenin, and chamomile is packed full of it. Apigenin, a potent antioxidant, is an inflammation prize fighter — just what you need to relieve those tender joints and foggy brain.

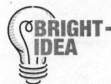

Spice up your meal with versatile chamomile

If you love it as a soothing hot tea, you'll be crazy about chamomile as a seasoning for your favorite foods. It has delicious flavors that make any meal special. Here are three ways to try it out.

- Ritzy rice. To add a mild, delicate fragrance to rice, hang used tea bags in a pot of water. Use fresh tea bags if you prefer a stronger chamomile flavor. When the water comes to a boil, remove the tea bags and add your rice, pasta, or other grains. Just take care when you're storing used bags. Refrigerate them in enough water to keep them wet. This prevents mold and the growth of bacteria.

- Kick'n chicken. Create a spice mix of chamomile — rub the flowers and leaves with your hands to break them up — and dried oregano, paprika, garlic, and lemon zest. Sprinkle evenly on the chicken and bake as desired.

- Mind-blowing homemade marinade. Use chamomile tea to flavor and tenderize meat. Bring 1/2 cup water to a boil and pour over four chamomile tea bags. Steep for 5 minutes and remove tea bags. Stir in 2 tablespoons extra-virgin olive oil, the juice from one lemon, 1 tablespoon honey, and salt and pepper. To tenderize meats, marinate in fridge for up to 24 hours.

Cherries

Food for thought — juice up your brain with this fantastic fruit

It was once illegal in Kansas to serve cherry pie with ice cream on top. Today you don't need to worry about the law, but the calories and sugar in this dessert should certainly give you second thoughts.

Why not opt for a simple glass of cherry juice instead? It's chock-full of flavor and brain-healthy antioxidants. You may find yourself wondering why you wanted pie a la mode in the first place.

Sweet cherries push back against dementia. Think of the last time you tried to learn something new — it required complex processes like language, attention, and memory to understand and use the information. But when you have dementia, these activities become much more difficult as the disease progresses.

Studies suggest that the flavonoids in berries may play a special role in keeping your brain healthy. Australian scientists have expanded on that research by testing whether cherries — which are rich in a type of flavonoid called anthocyanins — could improve cognitive function in people with dementia. Over 12 weeks the researchers gave 200 milliliters — about 3/4 cup a day — of either sweet Bing cherry juice or apple juice to seniors over age 70 with mild to moderate dementia.

The result? The cherry juice group showed improvements in verbal fluency — the ease at which they could remember information — as well as their short- and long-term memories. While cherry juice won't stop dementia from progressing, experts believe it may slow the loss of mental functions.

Improve brainpower and memory with tart cherries. A small University of Delaware study found that seniors who drank 1 cup of Montmorency tart cherry juice in the morning and at night over 12 weeks reacted faster and had fewer errors on cognitive function and memory tests than volunteers who drank a placebo. The cherry juice drinkers also felt more satisfied with their ability to remember information.

All the seniors were tested both before and after the trial on things like pattern recognition, information processing, and responses to visual cues on a screen.

Some families pass down recipes, others teach their children peculiar skills — like cherry-pit spitting. A Michigan family farm has held annual competitions for 45 years, drawing contestants from around the world who wanted to win the title of top cherry-pit spitter. While the last winner spat an impressive 54 feet, 3 inches, he couldn't beat the world record of nearly 94 feet.

Sheau Ching Chai, assistant professor of behavioral health and nutrition and lead researcher on the study, says the results may be due to tart cherries' ability to lower blood pressure. Several studies have linked high blood pressure to mental decline and memory problems.

"The potential beneficial effects of tart cherries may be related to the bioactive compounds they possess, which include polyphenols, anthocyanins, and melanin," she says.

Heard the juicy secret? Tart is smart for defending your health

Your first taste of tart cherry juice might be pleasantly surprising — it's not nearly as sour as you might expect. That's good news, because tart cherries may fend off a host of conditions like high blood pressure (BP), low-density lipoprotein (LDL) cholesterol, insomnia, and inflammation.

Raise a glass to a healthier heart. Studies have linked high cholesterol levels and BP to cardiovascular disease and a higher risk of developing dementia. But tart cherry juice — which is jam-packed with antioxidants, including proanthocyanins, anthocyanins, and flavonols — may lower both BP and cholesterol.

A 12-week study in *Food and Function* found that seniors who drank 1 cup of tart cherry juice in the morning and another at night had lower BP and LDL cholesterol than a control group. The researchers suggest compounds in tart cherries bind to bile acids, which helps clear LDL cholesterol from your system. All those antioxidants, meanwhile, are associated with improved blood vessel function and lower blood pressure.

Can't sleep? Phytochemicals bring relief. If you're worried about basic brainpower, catching enough ZZZs is essential. Sleep loss means sluggish reaction time, difficulty processing information, and a lousy mood. But sleeping pills are not the answer — try tart cherry juice instead. Some researchers believe a natural hormone in cherries called melatonin helps "shut off" your wakeful brain by signaling your body when it's time to sleep.

But other research suggests a phytochemical in tart cherry juice called procyanidin B2 may be doing the heavy lifting. In a small study, seniors with insomnia drank 1 cup of tart cherry juice in the morning and before bedtime every day for two weeks. Compared to a placebo group, their sleep time increased 84 minutes.

Researchers believe procyanidin B2 supresses an enzyme associated with inflammation and helps increase the availability of tryptophan, which contributes to better sleep quality.

Anti-inflammatories squash OA symptoms. Osteoarthritis (OA) is notorious for causing inflamed and painful joints. But a small study indicates tart cherry juice can lessen those symptoms. Participants with OA in the knee were randomly assigned to drink either two 8-ounce bottles of cherry juice or a placebo daily for six weeks.

Volunteers saw improvements in both knee pain and function while drinking the cherry juice. Their blood also had lower levels of high sensitivity C-reactive protein (hsCRP), an indicator of inflammation levels in your body. Studies suggest high levels of hsCRP may also increase the risk of dementia.

BRIGHT IDEA

Pit your cherries like a pro

Did you know you have over 1,000 varieties of cherries to choose from and every single one of them has a pit? Even the sweet little maraschino cherry is a stone fruit that somebody pitted for you. No need to let that stop you from enjoying these tasty and nutritious powerhouses. Check out these creative kitchen hacks for punching out cherry pits.

Before you start pitting, wash the cherries and take off their stems.

- Grab a small-necked bottle, a single chopstick, and your bowl of cherries. Place a cherry on top of the bottle opening and hold it between your fingers. Position the end of the chopstick on top of the cherry and push down. The seed should drop into the bottle.

- Stand a pastry tip on its flat end on a plate or cutting board. Gently push the cherry down onto the tip so the pit pops out.

- Pull the inner loop of a paperclip out at a right angle to form an L shape. Hold the cherry firmly between two fingers and insert the loop into the top of the cherry, rotate the clip, and scoop out the pit.

- Use clean tweezers to pluck out the pit as you hold the cherry between two fingers.

Don't toss your pits. Clean, dry, and store them until you have about a cup. They make the perfect filler for a DIY hot pack. Fashion a small pillow, fill it with the cherry pits, and microwave it in 30-second intervals to achieve the right temperature for you. Then place it on sore muscles or use for a headache.

Chewing gum

Chew on this: Improve concentration and fend off dementia for pennies

Folks around the world have enjoyed chewing gum for centuries. The ancient Aztecs even developed rules about when you could chew. For example, only kids and single women could chew in public. Men, married women, and widows indulged in secret. But these ancient gum chewers had no idea that chomping on this popular treat could keep their brains up to snuff. And it can still work for you.

A stick of gum can fine-tune your focus. A study looked at two groups of people who were told to listen to a series of numbers that were read in random order. Both groups were scored on how correctly and quickly they were able to pick out a series of odd-even numbers, like 7-2-1. The folks who chewed gum had quicker reaction times and better results than those who didn't chew gum, especially toward the end of the task.

"Participants who didn't chew gum performed slightly better at the beginning of the task but were overtaken by the end," says Kate Morgan, author of the study. "This suggests that chewing gum helps

When you were a kid, did you wonder what happened if you swallowed a piece of gum? Folklore told you it would stick in your stomach for seven years. Scary, but wrong. Your system can't digest gum base, but it easily passes through your system and is removed, just like other foods.

us focus on tasks that require continuous monitoring over a longer amount of time."

Chew your way to a better brain. Your brain relies on a constant flow of nutrition and oxygen to work at its best. But when your blood vessels can't supply what the brain needs, vascular dementia may develop. Researchers think the act of chewing makes more blood flow to the brain, and that may decrease your risk of dementia.

A study of 557 people, age 77 or older, showed that it didn't matter if folks chewed with their own natural teeth or with dentures. The researchers found that people who had difficulty chewing hard food were at a higher risk of developing cognitive problems. Now there's something to chew on, by gum!

Take a bite out of stress with a tasty chew

Oh, the delicious chewing gums of youth. Remember Fruit Stripe? Doublemint? How about Wrigley's Spearmint? You slipped a stick into your mouth before every math test, hoping the eagle-eyed teacher wouldn't see. You didn't know it then, but chewing on that tasty wad probably helped your algebra anxiety go way down. So will a couple of Chiclets still work to lower your stress today?

It seems almost unbelievable, but you can actually reduce fatigue, anxiety, and depression with a good chew. That's according to a study of more than 100 volunteers carried out at Cardiff University in Wales. And Japanese researchers from a separate study add one additional note — they discovered the harder you chew, the greater your stress relief. That study also said participants only had to chew for three minutes before their stress hormones went down.

So why does chewing gum work this way? Some parts of the brain like the hippocampus — the region in the brain that regulates your emotions and responds to stress — function differently when you're chewing. In fact, researchers think just the simple act of chewing may get the messenger cells in your hippocampus riled up enough to tamp down your stress and anxiety.

No need to look for a special gum. Any of your favorites will do the trick. Just sit back, relax, and chew away your stress.

Enjoy surprising perks in every pack

Baby shark, doo doo doo doo doo doo. Remember that song? One of the most annoying earworms — tunes that replay in your head in never-ending loops — of all time. Once it's in your brain, you can't get it out. At least, that's what you thought.

But now researchers have tracked volunteers who listened to music, and they discovered that folks who chewed gum reported one-third fewer earworms than their nonchewing counterparts. Experts say it may be because the gum chewing ties up the mental pathways used in imagining music. So what other perks do you get from chewing gum?

Are you feeling a little off-kilter? There's help. In one study, people with balance problems stood on a platform while researchers measured the amount of sway they displayed. Then the participants stood on the same platform, but this time they chewed gum for three minutes. The researchers observed much less swaying.

Go for gum to whittle your waist. Experts know being over-weight raises your risk of developing health problems linked to dementia like heart disease and type 2 diabetes. To help you get your weight under control, consider the power of gum.

Researchers studied the after-lunch appetites of 60 people to find out if chewing gum had any effect on their afternoon snacking habits. They found that popping a piece of chewing gum — regular or sugar-free — before snacking helped suppress appetite, block sweet cravings, reduce hunger, and decrease snacking by 36 calories. Every little bit helps.

Chew your way to a sparkling clean mouth. Just chomp on a stick of gum every day and you'll be armed to the teeth against harmful bacteria. Researchers say untreated dental infections can spread to your bloodstream and your brain. But if you chew gum just 10 minutes, that single piece of gum can remove 100 million bacteria in your saliva.

But be sure to choose sugarless gum. It turns out that gum with sugar could feed that oral bacteria you're trying to get rid of.

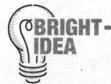

BRIGHT IDEA

Your gum's the real deal if you spot this seal

Ready to chew on some of those great gum benefits, but not sure which one to buy? The American Dental Association (ADA) has made your choice pretty simple — just keep an eye out for their seal.

All gums with the ADA Seal are sweetened with aspartame, sorbitol, mannitol, or other sweeteners that won't cause cavities. And that seal also tells you that the sugar-free gum has been tested in independent labs to prove it's safe and effective for reducing plaque and protecting tooth enamel.

For a list of approved sugar-free gums, check the ADA website at ada.org. You can find the Seal Product Search by clicking on "Seal of Acceptance" located under the Clinical Resources menu option.

Chocolate

3 cheers for chocolate — the snack that's packed with brain benefits

Do you know what chocolate has to do with the Nobel Prize? Believe it or not, a paper published in the *New England Journal of Medicine* suggests eating more chocolate may be linked to higher chances of winning the prestigious award.

Even if you're not trying to win a medal, experts say you have plenty of reasons to get more chocolate in your daily diet. In fact, cocoa may help you save your memory, fend of dementia, and even improve your mood.

Load up on cocoa to sharpen your memory. A study in the journal *Appetite* revealed that chowing down on chocolate could help beef up your brainpower. Researchers examined the diets of 968 people and gave them tests to measure cognitive abilities such as visual-spatial memory, word recall, reasoning, and attention. They discovered that the ones who ate chocolate at least once a week performed better than those who ate chocolate rarely or never.

The reason behind chocolate's brain-boosting benefits isn't completely clear yet, but experts think specific flavanols in cocoa beans help protect against normal age-related decline in mental skills.

Steer clear of dementia by snacking on chocolate. Portuguese researchers found the perfect excuse for chocolate lovers to reach for more cocoa. In a new study, they tracked the eating habits of over 530 seniors and discovered that eating more chocolate was linked to a lower risk of cognitive decline.

However, the experts said chocolate's protective powers were only seen in people who had less than 75 milligrams (mg) of caffeine every day, which is less than the amount in your morning cup of coffee. Keep in mind, a single ounce of dark chocolate alone has about 20 mg of caffeine.

Many scientists think compounds in the chocolate that give you a leg up against cognitive decline may one day also prove to protect against Alzheimer's disease.

Stressed? Soothe your mood with a sweet treat. A piece of chocolate can take the edge off after a long day. In a small study, researchers from the United Kingdom put chocolate's stress-fighting powers to the test.

They divided the participants into two groups. Half were given dark chocolate loaded with flavonoids, while others were given a control chocolate without these naturally occurring chemicals. After four weeks, those who ate the flavonoid-rich chocolate had lower levels of the stress hormone cortisol in their saliva.

> Shopping for cocoa powder? Avoid anything labeled "Dutched" or "processed with alkali." This process, which makes chocolate taste milder, also strips away the flavanols that give chocolate its health benefits. And if you're in the mood for a chocolate bar, aim for something that's at least 70% dark chocolate.

Want to try it yourself? People in the study ate 25 grams of dark chocolate every day. That's a bit less than you'd get in two half-ounce squares of baker's chocolate.

Call on cocoa to crush these common health concerns

Does your tin of cocoa powder belong in your medicine cabinet instead of the pantry? The ancient Aztecs probably thought so.

They treated infections with a drink brewed from cacao, also called cocoa beans, and tree bark.

Now, modern scientists are catching on to even more of chocolate's health benefits. Research shows that it can fight off stroke, heart disease, and diabetes.

Slash your risk of stroke by eating more of what you love. Strokes can be damaging within minutes, catastrophic within hours. Depending on what part of your brain is affected and for how long, memory, motor skills, speech, behavior, and thought processes can all be impaired. Fortunately, chocolate may help you avoid dangerous blood clots.

Researchers tracked the diets and health of more than 37,000 Swedish men for a decade. And after the scientists examined all the data, they found that those who ate the most chocolate had a 17% lower risk of stroke than those who didn't eat any at all.

How much did they eat? Around 63 grams of chocolate every week. That's a bit more than one bar of dark chocolate.

A few servings of chocolate could protect your ticker. Long-term studies have proved that the risk factors for heart disease also increase your chances of dementia. Fortunately, you might fend off both by unwrapping a chocolate bar.

Recently, experts examined the results of 23 studies that compared chocolate-eating habits to rates of heart events. And they discovered this delicious treat — about 45 grams a week — may be linked to a lower risk of heart disease.

The reason behind cocoa's heart-healthy benefits? Experts say the plant's flavanols help fight off inflammation, high blood pressure, and other risk factors.

This delicious dessert can help you dodge diabetes. A recent study found that seniors with type 2 diabetes may lose their memories more quickly than those without the condition. And while indulging in sweets is usually a bad idea when you're trying to ditch diabetes, experts think eating a couple of servings of chocolate every week could help you keep this dreaded disease at bay.

A new analysis published in *Nutrients* claims that eating one to six servings of chocolate every week can lower your risk of diabetes.

Be careful not to overdo it, though. Experts say you should keep your chocolate consumption to less than 100 grams — or about two bars of chocolate — a week, otherwise the sugar and calories could cancel out the health benefits.

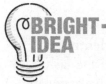

BRIGHT IDEA

Chocolate for dinner? Try these savory spins on a sweet treat

Who doesn't love a heaping scoop of chocolate ice cream? Or a chewy chocolate brownie? Of course, these sugar-laden desserts could undo the work of cocoa flavanols. Instead, consider adding a pinch of cocoa powder to your tomato soup or roasted chicken. It might sound strange, but chocolate has been used in savory dishes for centuries. Here are a few ways you can try it at home.

- Crunch on cocoa nibs. These broken bits of cocoa beans — which are used to make chocolate — add a nice crunch and bitterness to salads. And the best part? You get all the great benefits of chocolate without worrying about the sugar.

- Add a dash of unsweetened cocoa to sauces and stews. Pure, dark chocolate can add some depth to rich, acidic dishes. Next time you're making a batch of chili, put in a pinch of cocoa powder or 100% dark chocolate.

- Grate dark chocolate over your pasta. Italian cooks began adding chocolate to their dishes as soon as it arrived from the new world. Why? The bitter zing of chocolate cuts through cheesy pastas.

Coffee

Perk up your mind with a cup of joe

Coffee and clear thinking seem to go together. When Melitta Bentz got fed up tasting grounds in her morning coffee, she fashioned a filter from her son's blotting paper. She placed the paper in a tin pot and added coffee and boiling water. Voila! The daily grind of gritty coffee was over. Soon, the German housewife was producing filters for sale in her kitchen. More than 100 years later, the Melitta Group employs some 4,000 people. Now that's what clear thinking can do.

No matter how you drink it — caffeinated or decaffeinated — coffee does more than get your day started off right. Drinking 3 to 5 cups of this popular beverage every day could make you 65% less likely to develop Alzheimer's (AD) or other dementias in your later years.

Coffee cans the clumping that leads to AD. A jolt of java contains between 800 and 1,000 compounds — with caffeine being only one of them. Phenylindane is another and it may be helpful in preventing AD. Darker roasts of coffee appear to have higher concentrations of phenylindanes than lighter roasts.

Researchers at the University of Toronto believe phenylindane hinders the clustering of proteins called beta-amyloid and tau. Left unchecked, these proteins form plaques and tangles that can disrupt brain cell communication and lead to AD. The process can begin decades before any signs of dementia are obvious.

When the researchers investigated light, dark, and decaffeinated coffee extracts, they were surprised to find phenylindane — not caffeine — successfully blocked the accumulation of beta-amyloid. And it was better at preventing tau from clustering than any other compound they studied. This promising protective effect may be explained by phenylindane's surprisingly strong antioxidant capabilities.

Energize your mental and motor skills. Some studies indicate that coffee strengthens cognitive performance. Caffeine may be one of the reasons, but other research suggests there's more to it. Polyphenols called chlorogenic acids (CGAs), which you find more of in caffeinated coffee, may be at play.

To look at CGAs closer, two recent small studies evaluated seniors who drank beverages containing CGAs extracted from green coffee beans. Researchers found that CGAs may improve attention spans and executive function, the skills you need for organizing, structuring, and evaluating information. Improvements held true even among people with mild cognitive impairment (MCI), as was the case in one of the studies published in the *Journal of Alzheimer's Disease*.

Among other reasons, the antioxidants in CGAs are thought to protect neurons and block beta-amyloid buildup. That effect could improve vascular function in the brain and possibly encourage nerve growth.

The latest scoop: Drink java to drop health risks

American colonists first tasted coffee in New Amsterdam — part of present-day New York City — in the 1600s. But coffee played second fiddle to tea until the Boston Tea Party. Once patriots found they could ditch the highly taxed British tea for this pick-me-up, they were hooked.

As are the people today. The U.S. coffee industry is currently worth about $48 billion. But the brew has much more to offer than a colorful history. Many flock to cafes for social gatherings, conversation, or study time. But others turn to coffee for its promising health perks.

Coffee keeps your heart healthy. Calcium deposits, a part of artery-clogging plaque, have been linked to a higher risk of heart attack, stroke, and dementia. But a tasty latte could brew up some benefits.

In the Rotterdam Coronary Calcification Study, researchers used a noninvasive, sensitive scanning tool called electron beam computed tomography to measure calcium levels inside the coronary arteries of 1,570 Dutch adults between the ages of 55 and 86.

The men and women also reported how much coffee they drank in a typical week. The results? Women who drank 3 or more cups a day were less likely to have severe calcium buildup in their arteries than women who drank less than that. The researchers say phytoestrogens in coffee may replace declining levels of the heart-healthy hormone estrogen after menopause.

> Leave out the sugary concoctions and your coffee might help you prevent cavities. Experts say people who enjoy about 3 cups of medium-roasted, black coffee a day get the added perk of strong antioxidant protection in their mouths. Coffee may also cut down on plaque and help control inflammation of the gums.

Dial back your diabetes risk. Findings from three large U.S. studies — the Nurses' Health Study (NHS), NHS II, and the Health Professionals Follow-up Study — reveal a preventive role for caffeinated coffee when it comes to diabetes.

Researchers found that adults who drank more than 1 extra cup of coffee a day over a four-year period had an 11% lower risk of developing type 2 diabetes than those who made no changes to the amount they drank. Those who cut back on their coffee by more than 1 cup during the same period had a 17% greater risk of developing the disease.

Why is avoiding diabetes important for your brain? High blood sugar can damage your blood vessels, which can result in poor blood circulation to your brain. That can make it difficult to think clearly.

If you already have type 2 diabetes, talk to your doctor about your coffee consumption. Research suggests the caffeine in coffee causes some people with the disease to experience spikes in blood sugar and insulin levels.

BRIGHT IDEA

Add in flavor, ditch extra calories

Have you heard of the latest craze of adding butter and coconut oil to coffee? Although the concoction may have a creamy rich taste, 2 tablespoons of each ingredient in your morning brew contain a hefty 445 calories. You'd have to chop wood for an hour to burn that off.

The happy truth is you have more choices than ever when it comes to flavoring your coffee. That makes it easy to liven up your cup without extra calories or fat. Take a look at how traditional options stack up against more healthy alternatives.

Flavor	Amount	Calories	Fat (grams)
stevia	1/4 teaspoon	0	0
unsweetened cocoa powder	1 teaspoon	4	0.2
cardamom	1 teaspoon	6.2	0.1
cinnamon	1 teaspoon	6.2	0
nutmeg	1 teaspoon	10.5	0.7
powdered creamer	1 teaspoon	10.9	0.7
vanilla extract	1 teaspoon	11.5	0
milk, 1%	1 ounce	12.8	0.3
sugar	1 teaspoon	15.5	0
agave nectar	1 teaspoon	21	0
half-and-half	1 ounce	39	3.4
maple syrup	1 tablespoon	52.2	0
liquid creamer	1 ounce	58.5	5.8
honey	1 tablespoon	63.8	0

Cooking

2 ways to cook up brain-healthy benefits

Hate to cook? You're not alone — a recent survey found that 45% of Americans can't stand spending time in the kitchen. But some new data might change your mind. This everyday chore can improve your brainpower and your mood.

Hone your kitchen skills to sharpen your mind. If you've ever been tasked with hosting a holiday dinner, you know that cooking a half-dozen dishes at once is a mental workout. You have to make sure the turkey hits the table right at 6, exactly when the rolls are ready. And you need to watch the veggies so they don't burn, all while keeping an eye on the potatoes to keep them from overboiling.

Even though hosting Thanksgiving seems exhausting, experts think that taking charge on these meals could help keep your mind in tiptop shape. Researchers divided 57 healthy seniors into two groups and tested them on their cognitive abilities. Half of the seniors then participated in five weekly computer-assisted sessions where they were required to properly time the cooking of several foods. As a secondary task, they "virtually" set as many tables as possible.

The control group didn't participate in such activities. At the completion of the study, all of the seniors were once again tested on their cognitive abilities. The scientists found that the people in the cooking group showed improvements in their working memory, an executive function that controls how you process, use, and remember information.

Feeling stressed? Whip up a meal. Few things are more relaxing after a long day than eating a tasty and nutritious home-cooked dinner. Researchers now think making a nice meal could help improve your mood, too.

In a recent review, experts examined the results of 11 studies about the benefits of cooking. The data showed that learning to cook can improve self-esteem and quality of life. And senior women with dementia who cooked under strict supervision decreased their levels of agitation, too.

The authors weren't sure why cooking led to these improvements, but they have a couple of theories. Cooking can help improve cognitive function, and that may bring about improvements in depression and anxiety. And cooking can also make it easier to eat healthy foods that brighten your mood.

3 strategies for fending off food poisoning

Can't tell if that milk in your fridge smells sour? As you age, your sense of taste and smell starts to fade. That can make it hard to tell if your food is still safe to eat. And seniors often have less stomach acid and a weaker immune system, which means they are at risk for food-borne illnesses. Here's how you can stay safe.

- Keep perishables in the fridge. If you're thawing frozen foods, don't do it at room temperature. And if you use the microwave to defrost food, cook it immediately.

- Can't eat all of your takeout? You shouldn't leave food out at room temperature for more than two hours. If you're storing hot food, divide it into smaller portions and only reheat what you're going to eat.

- Use a food thermometer. You can find one at your local grocery store. These tools are great for making sure meat cooks at a safe temperature.

Use your kitchen to dodge these dreaded conditions

Experts say ordering restaurant delivery is five times more expensive than cooking your meals at home. And home-cooked dinners aren't just cheaper. They're healthier, too — if you do it right.

Home-cooked meals help you lose weight. If you're overweight, you're more likely to have higher levels of a specific protein called C-reactive protein (CRP). And CRP is associated with thinking and memory problems, as well as dementia. If you want to shed those extra pounds, the best place to start is in the kitchen.

Researchers at Johns Hopkins University analyzed data from a large nutrition survey and found

Want to get more hands-on experience in the kitchen? Consider taking a senior-specific cooking class. Your local senior center or community college may offer cooking courses that teach you how to eat healthier, use food bank staples, and make sure your meals last throughout the month.

that people who frequently cooked at home ate fewer calories than people who cooked less often. That's probably because food eaten outside the home — at a drive-thru, for example — tends to have more fat and sugar, the researchers say. What's more, those who frequently cooked made healthier choices when they ate out.

Turn down the heat to heal your heart. What you cook is only part of the battle. Believe it or not, how you cook your meals might help you avoid heart disease. And experts say lowering the risk of heart disease could help you keep your mind sharp, too.

A new study in *Nutrition* revealed high-heat cooking methods — such as frying and roasting — create trans-fatty acids and other toxic chemical compounds that may increase your risk of heart disease. Try steaming, poaching, and boiling your foods to avoid these dangerous chemicals.

Breathe easy when you opt to grill. Experts say your brain needs 20% of all the oxygen you breathe. So it shouldn't surprise you that research suggests chronic lung disease can increase your risk of dementia.

Now scientists think your cooking fuel can increase your risk of breathing problems. A study of 280,000 Chinese adults who never smoked found that those who cooked with wood or coal were at a higher risk of being hospitalized or dying from respiratory disease than people who used gas or electricity.

While most Americans don't use a wood-burning stove in their home, it's probably a good idea to be mindful of the type of fuel you use when grilling out. Consider using natural gas or propane instead of charcoal or smoking woods.

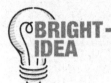

BRIGHT IDEA

Stay safe in the kitchen — tips to help you handle the heat

Cooking is a great way to keep your mind focused and protect your health. But you still need to be careful in the kitchen. Sharp knives, hot stoves, and slippery floors could be dangerous for seniors. Fortunately, a few simple tweaks can help you avoid accidents.

- Put anti-slip flooring in the kitchen. Most falls occur here and in the bathroom.

- Install extra lighting. Make sure you can see everything, so you don't lose bits of food, cut yourself, or slip on something.

- Keep a timer on hand. Set it whenever you're cooking, so you don't forget about food in the oven or on the stove.

- Watch out for fire hazards. Keep curtains, towels, and potholders away from the stove. And avoid wearing loose-fitting sleeves while you're cooking.

However, if you or a loved one has dementia, cooking alone might not be a good idea. Even with safety tools in place, the risk of cuts, burns, falls, and fires is too high.

Dairy

It does a body good: Maintain your mind with milk and dairy

Want to get your money's worth out of that carton of milk? Add a dash of table salt or baking soda and give yourself another week to enjoy it. But how to buy your brain precious time against memory loss and dementia? Milk and dairy could be key.

Dairy dials back dementia risk. Folks who sport milk mustaches can feel good about defending their health against serious conditions — like high blood pressure, diabetes, obesity, and stroke — that also pave the way for dementia. That's one explanation researchers gave for their encouraging results from a 17-year study of the diet and health of Japanese people age 60 and older.

> The natural yellow color of butter comes mainly from beta carotene found in the grass cows eat. Cow's milk isn't yellow because the fat membranes haven't been broken. But when that milk or cream is churned for butter, fat membranes break and color is exposed. Butter from pasture-grazing bovine is a brighter yellow in spring and summer.

They found that participants who ate or drank more dairy or milk had a significantly lower risk of developing dementia, particularly Alzheimer's disease.

Dairy provides key nutrients like calcium, magnesium, vitamin B12, and whey protein — all of which play a role in protecting your brain.

Make the most of your memory. Forget where you put your keys — again? No doubt about it, short-term memory comes in handy. Fortunately, men who eat and drink more dairy products appear to perform better on story recall — a test of short-term memory — according to a twin study published in *Clinical Nutrition*. This finding was consistent with other studies and may be due to dairy's B12 and calcium.

The same results were not seen in women, but, ladies, don't count out the power of vitamin D found in fortified dairy products. In one study, researchers asked senior women with low vitamin D levels to eat yogurt fortified with calcium and vitamin D or unfortified yogurt every day for three months. The group that ate the fortified yogurt performed better on tests that measure attention, memory, language, and visual-spatial skills.

Calcium supplements call for caution

Milk a cow twice a day and you'll get about 10 gallons of milk daily — that's 160 glasses of milk. By that cow culation you should have plenty of milk available, so you might not need to resort to calcium supplements. That's good news because supplements can be risky for certain people.

Adults begin to lose bone mass after their 30s, which is the reason you need calcium — to maintain as much bone mass as possible. But supplements may not be the best way to get it for everyone, according to a study published in *Neurology*.

The researchers examined women with a history of cerebrovascular disease, which includes conditions — like stoke, ministroke, and aneurysm — that interfere with the brain's blood supply. The women who took calcium supplements were twice as likely to develop dementia compared to those who did not take them.

Fortunately, the calcium you get through a variety of foods appears to protect against vascular problems.

Dairy on the daily: To rev up your health eat more of these foods

In a sketch by American cartoonist Leo Cullum, a chicken asks her friend, the cow, "Milk, butter, cheese? Aren't you spreading yourself a bit thin?" The chicken makes a good point. Milk is versatile enough to find its way into dozens of dairy products. And while you're enjoying those tasty foods, don't forget to appreciate the many ways they keep you healthy and strong throughout life.

- Deny diabetes. Your blood vessels are like the first domino in a chain. Diabetes can damage them, putting you at risk for vascular dementia. This type of dementia occurs from the brain damage caused by blocked blood flow to your brain. Low-fat dairy and yogurt has been associated with a reduced risk of diabetes.

- Bet on better blood pressure. Pop quiz! What's a leading cause of stroke? That's right — high blood pressure. It can have devastating effects on your brain. But folks with low calcium could see an improvement in their blood pressure by getting the recommended amount of calcium daily, whether it be through dairy or supplements.

- Value your vision. When you can't see very well, your ability to participate in activities that stimulate your brain is limited. Although more study is needed, researchers found that dietary calcium and calcium supplements are associated with a lower risk of developing late age-related macular degeneration.

- Maintain muscles. Frailty and sarcopenia are both characterized by lost strength and muscle mass. And both can lead to falls that cause injury. Sarcopenia may also cause delirium and is closely linked to Alzheimer's disease.

  Studies show that low levels of vitamin D in older people are related to loss of muscle mass and strength. But seniors have shown improvements in muscle strength by supplementing this sunshine vitamin.

• Ward off weight gain. Conditions arising from obesity, including diabetes, high blood pressure, and heart disease, can be a bane for your brain. Women with normal weight who ate or drank high-fat, or whole, dairy products and milk were less likely to put on extra weight over an average of 11 years in the Women's Health Study.

Strangely enough, these weight loss results did not hold true for low-fat dairy. Researchers explained their finding lined up with other studies, but notably they excluded data from women who were already obese at the beginning of the study.

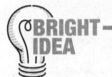

BRIGHT IDEA

Get powerful nutrients from plant-based milks

Regular milk is a champ when it comes to brain-boosting and disease-preventing nutrition. But plant-based milk alternatives stand ready to take up the fight for your health, too. In the arena of milk alternatives, look for fortified options first. They can deliver a knockout when it comes to key vitamins and minerals. See how a cup of these milks stack up against the others.

Type	Calories	Fat (grams)	Calcium (%DV*)	Vitamin B12 (%DV*)	Vitamin D (%DV*)
almond	40	3	35	25	0
coconut	50	5	10	50	30
goat	140	7	30	0	25
pea	70	4.5	35	100	30
rice	120	2	30	25	25
soy	80	4	20	120	15

*Percent daily value (%DV) is the percentage of the recommended daily amount found in a serving of the food, based on a 2,000-calorie diet for healthy adults.

Dancing

Take a bow: Dancing can improve your brain function

"Dance even if you have nowhere to do it but your living room," says famed Chicago Tribune columnist Mary Schmich. And she's right. Light exercise can improve your health. Just take five hours out of your week — a little more than 40 minutes a day — to trip the light fantastic. You'll twirl your way to better brain health, no problem.

Cut a rug to slow brain volume loss. The hippocampus is your brain's center for memory, learning, and balance. You can keep it fit with physical exercise, and dance's benefits are "on point" when it comes to reversing brain aging.

Alzheimer's disease and normal aging can damage this part of your brain. In fact, it's possible to lose 2% to 3% of your hippocampus over a decade. This neuron loss can speed up after you turn 70. But recent research suggests you can outpace this damage with a quick two-step.

A German study published in *Frontiers in Human Neuroscience* examined the brain volume of 52 healthy seniors who either practiced new dance routines or participated in flexibility and strength-endurance training. They all exercised for 90 minutes, twice a week for six months and then once a week for another 12 months.

Dr. Kathrin Rehfeld, lead author of the study, says, "In this study, we show that two different types of physical exercise (dancing and endurance training) both increase the area of the brain that declines with age." That area of the brain is the hippocampus. But the dancers bagged an added bonus — they showed volume growth in more areas of the hippocampus.

Don your dancing shoes for a brighter mood. "Happy feet! I've got those happy feet!" sings Bing Crosby in a lively number from the 1930 film "The King of Jazz." Good thing too, because studies suggest that the exercise you get in activities like dancing can improve your mood.

Researcher Weiyun Chen, who analyzed data from 23 studies on happiness and physical activity, found that, "Even a small change of physical activity makes a difference in happiness." Some of the studies suggested that people who were "sufficiently active" were nearly 30% more likely to be happy than inactive people.

But how active you are only matters to a point. The researchers found that happiness levels were the same in people who worked out between 2 1/2 and five hours a week and those who exercised more than five hours a week.

Why is being happy important to your brain health? Depression can affect your ability to focus, making it difficult to remember things.

Ease Parkinson's symptoms with the tango. It takes two to tango, but the benefits of this dance are all yours. As researchers at McGill University in Canada found out, the tango may help treat the symptoms of Parkinson's disease (PD).

They divided 40 men and women with PD into two groups. Over the course of 12 weeks, one set learned to tango in professionally taught classes. The other participated in a self-directed exercise group. At the end of the study, the researchers found that the dancers showed significant improvements in balance and mobility. The scientists say the tango's rhythmic forward and backward stepping patterns may

Learning to dance in the comfort of your home is as easy as turning on your computer. Just search "dance lessons for seniors/beginners" at *youtube.com* for hours of simple routines. Looking for a specific style? Try "Learn to square dance," or whatever fits your fancy, and break out your jazz hands.

be particularly helpful when it comes to walking difficulties in people with PD.

The dancers also showed improved cognitive function. One possible reason? You need to multitask, pay attention, and use your working memory to get all the movements right, step to the beat, and avoid bumping into others on the dance floor.

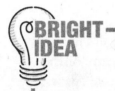

BRIGHT IDEA

Protect yourself from injury with these tips

"Dance first. Think later. It's the natural order," goes a famous misquote from a play by Samuel Beckett. It may sound like good advice for a carefree life, but the exact opposite is true when you're getting ready to trip the light fantastic. So take these precautions to avoid injury.

Prior to even attempting a pirouette, talk to your doctor about any medical conditions that may stop you from dancing. If you have the go-ahead, it's time to get footloose. Kick off your Sunday shoes and swap them for appropriate footwear — the wrong shoes can cause blisters, bruising, and ingrown toenails.

While you're picking out your outfit, stick to comfortable, well-fitting clothing. Layers may be your best bet because you can shed a few as you warm up — a pre-workout step you should always do.

And before you really get moving, make sure you nosh on a snack so you have enough energy to get groovin' — staying hydrated is key, too, so keep a water bottle with you.

Take a break if you need it and don't push yourself too hard. You run the risk of hurting yourself more through overtraining, fatigue, and failing to rest injuries.

If you're in a class setting, keep an eye on your instructor, classmates, and even yourself to keep your form in shape and troubleshoot your challenges. Poor technique and posture is an injury risk in dance.

Tap into the heart-healing, balance-renewing powers of dance

A little dance will do ya when it comes to choreographing a plan to revitalize your health. Whether you're down to cha cha across the room or prefer a neat jazz square, dance may be the two-step you need to better your heart and balance.

Kick up your heels and keep heart disease at bay. Sometimes light footwork doesn't cut it. In a survey of more than 48,000 adults over age 40, researchers found that moderate-intensity, but not light-intensity, dancing and walking were linked to lower rates of death from cardiovascular disease.

Heart disease spells trouble for your brain. It can damage your blood vessels and interfere with the steady supply of oxygen-rich blood to your brain. But you can reduce your risk of dying from heart disease with moderate- or high-intensity dance — it works even better than walking.

So how can you tell if you're exercising hard enough? You'll get sweaty and feel out of breath if you've reached moderate-intensity dancing. Some dance styles even mirror high intensity interval training, and may include short vigorous spurts of activity followed by light-intensity dancing. That kind of a workout appears to offer more cardiovascular benefits than continuous training.

Looking for better balance? Get down and boogie. In "It's a Wonderful Life," George Bailey and Mary Hatch dance the Charleston across the gym floor, skirting the brink of the pool opening up beneath their feet. Although this beloved duo eventually lost their balance and tumbled into the water, you don't have to. Without pools to disrupt your fancy footwork, dance can do wonders for your balance.

In the story *Take a bow: Dancing can improve your brain function*, the study analyzing endurance training and dancing showed both activities had an anti-aging effect on the brain. But according to lead researcher Kathrin Rehfeld, "It was only dancing that led to noticeable behavioral changes in terms of improved balance."

The dance lessons mixed foundational movements like head-spins and weight shifts with classic steps like chassée, mambo, and grapevine to challenge the participants' balance skills. The seniors who danced improved their balance, which is important as you age to prevent falls that can lead to broken bones and loss of independence.

Improving your balance can help you keep your independence in other ways, too. In an eight-year study of women between the ages of 75 and 84, researchers found that those who danced were were more likely to independently perform activities of daily living — walking, eating, bathing, dressing, and using the bathroom — than their nondancing peers. The scientists say the balance, strength, endurance, and focus needed to dance may help keep your brain young and keep you self-reliant.

4 questions to find the jig that's right for you

Ready to start dancing? Ask yourself these questions to help you decide which style of dance to try.

- What kind of music do you enjoy? If you like country songs, zydeco, or bluegrass music, square dancing may be for you. If you love swing, music from past decades, or Latin music, you might try ballroom dance.

- Would you rather dance alone, with a partner, or as part of a group? Ballroom dance, for instance, requires a partner, but you can participate in any line dance without one.

- Are classes available in your area, or can you be happy learning from a video? A local hula instructor may be tough to find.

- What type of dance have you always dreamed of trying? Pick one you're really interested in. If you're motivated by a true love of the dance, you'll be more inclined to stick with it.

DASH diet

Make a DASH for a sharper brain and brighter mood

Nutrisystem. South Beach. Jenny Craig. Just three of the famous weight loss plans endorsed by flashy celebrities. And if you stick to their strict menus, you could lose some weight. But what if you found a diet that could help you drop a few pounds — without restricting your food choices? Not only that, but this plan sharpens your brain, lowers blood pressure, and even decreases depression. Sound good? It's called the DASH diet, and now is the time to learn all about it. No celebrities needed.

The letters in DASH stand for dietary approaches to stop hypertension. If you eat about 2,000 calories a day, your daily menu will look something like this.

- four to five servings each of fruits and vegetables

- six to eight servings of whole grains

- six or fewer servings of fish, poultry, and lean meat

- two to three servings of dairy

You can also enjoy four to five servings of nuts, seeds, and legumes every week. Even occasional sweets. Is your mouth watering yet?

Sustain your brain by lowering your blood pressure. The DASH diet's main goal is to keep your blood pressure in check. And that's important because high blood pressure can cause your arteries to become stiff and narrow, limiting blood flow to your brain. This can lead to vascular dementia, which involves problems with reasoning, planning, judgment, and memory.

An 11-year study of nearly 4,000 people over age 65 showed that the closer someone followed the DASH plan, the better their scores were on cognitive tests. The researchers also found that four of the DASH diet's food groups were superstars when it came to cognitive function, those mental abilities that include learning, reasoning, and remembering. So focus on the big four — vegetables, whole grains, low-fat dairy, and nuts or legumes.

The DASH diet derails depression. Research shows folks who eat vegetables, fruits, and grains may have a lower risk of developing depression over time than people who follow a more Western-style diet with lots of saturated fats and red meats.

"Making a lifestyle change such as changing your diet is often preferred over taking medications, so we wanted to see if diet could be an effective way to reduce the risk of depression," said Dr. Laurel Cherian of Rush University Medical Center in Chicago.

For the study, almost 1,000 people with an average age of 81 were evaluated every year for more than six years. They were divided into three groups based on how well they stuck to the DASH diet. The two groups that followed the diet most closely were less likely to develop depression than the people in the group who didn't closely follow it. In fact, the odds of becoming depressed over time was 11% lower among top DASH followers compared to the lowest group.

Looking for a sharper memory and better learning and reasoning skills? Less depression? Then it's time to make the DASH to a better brain.

DASH diet too tough to follow? Simply make changes to your regular menu, and — voila! — you'll be a DASHer in no time. Treat meat as one part of your meal — not the main dish — and try to cut large portions by half. Use fruit as desserts and snacks. Fresh, dried, or fruit canned in their own juice are good choices.

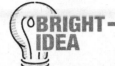

Table the salt to ease the pressure

Your blood pressure rises and falls during the day. That's normal. But if it stays too high for too long, you have high blood pressure (HBP). HBP makes your heart work harder, and that hurts your arteries. HBP can lead to heart disease, kidney disease — even stroke.

And salt is a big part of the problem. In the standard DASH diet, you can have no more than 2,300 milligrams (mg) of sodium each day — about 1 teaspoon of table salt. And if you have high blood pressure, DASH suggests you keep your intake below 1,500 mg. Need a little help shaking the extra salt out of your diet?

Beware sodium's game of hide-and-seek. Here's a quiz for you. Which pantry staple has the most sodium? Two pork sausage links or half a cup of instant vanilla pudding? Surprise! It's the pudding, with 350 mg of sodium. The sausage links? A close 310 mg. Dodge hidden salt with these tips.

- Read the labels.

- Eat more fresh fruits and vegetables.

- Rinse canned foods like beans and tuna.

- Flavor your food with herbs like oregano, cilantro, rosemary, and thyme.

Make smart plans for an evening out. It's Mom's birthday, and she always chooses Italian for her special dinner. Yikes. How will you stick to DASH?

- Visit the restaurant's website to check out the sodium count on your favorite menu items. You can also search for your dish on *calorieking.com*. The site includes nutrition data from hundreds of restaurants nationwide.

- Steer clear of foods that are pickled, cured, or contain soy sauce.

- Skip condiments like mustard, ketchup, and pickles. And push the salt shaker away.

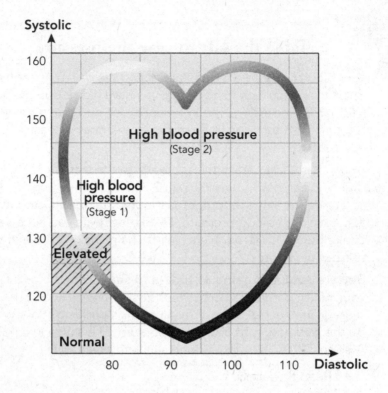

Appetizing extras: Crush cholesterol and ditch diabetes

"Whatever your problem is, the answer is not in the fridge," goes a popular saying. The point of the proverb is to curb emotional eating. But if you struggle with high cholesterol or blood sugar, the answer may very well be in your refrigerator — so long as you're sticking to the DASH diet.

Drop cholesterol numbers to up your heart health. DASH is famous for tackling high blood pressure, but it also helps your heart in other ways — like fighting off high cholesterol. This is important for your brain, too. Researchers have found that high levels of LDL cholesterol (often called bad cholesterol) paired with low levels of HDL cholesterol (also known as the good kind) are linked to having more amyloid plaques in the brain, which may contribute to Alzheimer's disease.

Ready to balance your cholesterol levels to protect your brain and lower your risk of heart disease? DASH could do it for you. Here's how.

- First, you get lots of fiber from fruits and veggies, whole grains, nuts, and beans. Fiber lowers your LDL by attaching to the cholesterol particles and keeping them from entering your bloodstream.

- Next, you eat plenty of fish and leaner cuts of meat which help reduce your triglycerides, the most common type of fat in the body. High levels of triglycerides increase your risk of developing heart disease.

- Finally, you limit sweets, refined carbs, and saturated fats. Swapping those for healthy fats and whole grains is linked to better triglyceride, LDL, and HDL levels.

Diabetes is no match for DASH. Diabetes can damage your blood vessels over time. That includes the small blood vessels in the brain. This damage affects your brain's white matter, putting you at risk for vascular dementia.

Two out of 3 people with type 2 diabetes also have high blood pressure. So it seems like the DASH diet would be a good fit for folks battling both. In a study of 31 people with type 2 diabetes, the DASH plan improved blood pressure while lowering A1C — their estimated average glucose over the past few months — by almost 2 percentage points.

And a meta-analysis shows that the DASH diet was associated with a 20% decrease in the risk of developing type 2 diabetes in the future. Given the health benefits of the DASH plan, along with its recommendation to eat many different kinds of healthy foods, researchers say the DASH diet may be just the thing for folks fighting type 2 diabetes.

Deep breathing

Harness the powers of breathing to sustain your brain

Breathing is one of the most basic functions of human life and comes so naturally that you may take it for granted. But that leaves money, or in this case health benefits, on the table. Channel your breathing to put wind in the sails of your attention span and mood — all you have to do is focus and inhale.

Breathe new life into your attention span. Low and high levels of noradrenaline — a chemical messenger in your brain — can make it harder to focus. But hitting the perfect level helps you think clearer and encourages your brain to grow new connections. Can you influence noradrenaline production? Yes, say scientists, by mastering your breathing.

While studying the locus coeruleus, the part of the brainstem where most of your noradrenaline is made, researchers at Trinity College Dublin found a link between breathing patterns and focus. Participants who focused well during an attention-demanding task had better synchronization between their breathing patterns and their attention, compared to those with poor focus.

"This study has shown that as you breathe in locus coeruleus activity is increasing slightly, and as you breathe out it decreases," says Michael Melnychuk, lead author of the study. "Put simply this means that our attention is influenced by our breath and that it rises and falls with the cycle of respiration. It is possible that by focusing on and regulating your breathing you can optimize your attention level."

The study examined two types of breath-focused practices that you can try out yourself to tame your wandering mind.

- For a concentration boost, put mindful breathing to the test. Focus on how your breath flows in and out without trying to control it.

- With pranayama, on the other hand, practice controlling your breath. Sometimes you're not focused because you're either not stimulated enough — think drowsy driving — or because you're overstimulated — think nerves during a public speech. This is when controlled breathing may be most helpful.

> YAWNNN. Time to hit the hay? Not necessarily. Yawning can be a sign of what you're feeling, like tiredness, but it has other uses, too. It may even act as your brain's personal cooling system by increasing blood flow in your neck and head, and pulling cool air into your mouth, which cools the blood traveling to your brain.

Combat stress with the relaxation response. This state of deep rest can change how you react to stress both physically and emotionally. Your heart beat slows, blood pressure drops, and muscles relax.

To reap the benefits, you may think you just have to sit still and wait. But relaxing actually requires active work, and the key is focused breathing. Just 20 to 30 minutes of abdominal breathing each day can reduce anxiety and stress, according to The American Institute of Stress.

Abdominal breathing is a technique often used when practicing yoga. One type — involving rhythmic breaths moving through slow, medium, and fast cycles — can reduce depression in addition to stress and anxiety.

Deep breathing boosts your brain's oxygen supply and turns on the parasympathetic nervous system, which creates a feeling of relaxation. It also triggers the longest cranial nerve, called the vagus nerve, to release chemicals that have a calming effect on the body. All this leaves you in tune with your body and out of your head and its worries.

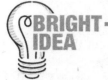

Renew and restore: 2 techniques you can start now

Breathe in. Breathe out. It sounds simple enough, but there's more than one way to fill up your lungs. With these two practices, don't aim for perfection. Focus on gentle and unforced air flow. Over time your efforts will be paid back with health benefits.

Abdominal breathing. Also called diaphragmatic or belly breathing, this technique teaches you to breathe from your belly instead of your chest, which adds strain to your neck and shoulders.

- Start in a comfortable position, sitting down or lying on your back.

- Rest one hand on your upper chest and the other on your stomach, just below your rib cage.

- Slowly, take a breath through your nose. The hand on your stomach should move as your diaphragm pushes out while the other remains relatively still.

- Exhale through pursed lips, focusing on your abdomen pushing inward.

- Continue this breathing technique for five to 10 minutes.

Alternate-nostril breathing. This breath pattern takes more concentration than abdominal breathing because you're using your fingers, too. Let your breath pull your attention away from your thoughts.

- Start by sitting in a comfortable position with your left hand on your left knee.

- Close your right nostril by pressing with your right thumb.

- Take a breath through your left nostril.

- Using your right index finger close your left nostril, then remove your thumb from your right.

- Exhale through your right nostril.

- Inhale then close the right nostril again with your thumb.

- Remove your index finger from the left side and exhale.

- Continue this pattern for up to five minutes.

Draw in a trio of perks with focused breathing

The vast benefits of controlling your breathing pattern might knock the wind out of you. Exercises that adapt your breathing style offer a multitude of blessings, from a good night's sleep to better blood pressure, so take in the breath of life and get going.

Breathe out bad vibes for better sleep. Concerned about brainpower? Catching enough ZZZs is fundamental. Losing sleep could lead to slower reaction times, trouble making decisions, difficulty processing information, and more negative emotions.

When stress stops you from getting enough shut-eye, shift your attention to your breathing. As you lie in bed, let your mind concentrate on each inhale and exhale. Pinpoint areas of tension in your body and relax — releasing that tightness when you breathe out can help you fall asleep.

Push out pain with each exhale. Chronic pain can cause changes in brain activity that are linked to depression, anxiety, and difficulty making decisions. But focused breathing could offer relief. It redirects your attention away from whatever ache is ailing you. This eases up the stress and tension that can make your pain even worse.

Plus researchers have found that breathing exercises can improve lung function, reduce back pain, and improve quality of life. With only four to eight weeks of regular practice needed to bag these benefits, perfecting your breathing is a safe and easy way to take control of your pain at home.

Slow breaths ease blood pressure. Research has linked high blood pressure (HBP) to memory loss and a reduced ability to think quickly. But you may be able to stop it from bursting your thought bubbles with deep breathing.

Slowing to 10 breaths or fewer per minute is enough to lower blood pressure in some people. This pacing can calm your sympathetic nervous system, which is in charge of fight or flight responses and regulates important functions such as blood pressure.

Adding a listening cue like music may help you get as low as five breaths per minute. That's what happened for some participants in a recent study. They were given a CD to guide their breathing with one sound to prompt inhalation and another for exhalation. The researchers following their progress found that after eight weeks, this music-guided deep breathing reduced blood pressure in participants with HBP.

The real reason you sigh (and what it means for your health)

Whoosh. Out flows a sigh of frustration, boredom, or even relief. And with that simple action, you've revitalized your lungs.

The tiny air sacs in your lungs called alveoli are in charge of passing oxygen and carbon dioxide molecules between your lungs and bloodstream. But they can collapse during normal breathing. As large breaths — some two to five times the size of a normal breath — sighs may re-expand those air sacs and bring your breathing back to normal.

In addition, a study published in *Biological Psychology* found that taking a deep breath gave participants relief after they faced a series of positive and negative images. Why? When you experience strong emotions like fear and anxiety, your body disrupts its normal breathing cycle while trying to increase oxygen flow. Sighing is like pressing the reset button, helping you return to healthy breathing patterns.

Dental hygiene

Operation clean mouth: Fight plaque to save your brain

Bad breath may keep folks out of your personal space, but it could also be a warning sign. Let food build up between your gums and teeth and you'll eventually have more than odor in your mouth. You'll see tartar — an accumulation of hardened plaque — around your gum line.

In the early stage of gum disease called gingivitis, that buildup of plaque may eventually cause your gums to bleed easily and become red and puffy. Left untreated, gingivitis turns into an infection that is tough to fight. It can even endanger your health. In fact, research suggests that gum disease may be at the root of Alzheimer's disease (AD). And poor dental health could be tied to declines in mental health as you age.

Bacteria tip the balance toward AD. The bacteria *Porphyromonas (P.) gingivalis* is the lead bad guy when it comes to the most serious form of gum disease, periodontitis. And a team of researchers now believe it may play a role in the development of AD.

They compared brain samples of deceased people with and without AD who were about the same age when they died. The scientists found that the brains of the people with AD had significantly higher levels of toxins produced by *P. gingivalis*.

How did the toxins get there? The researchers studied mice injected with *P. gingivalis* and found that the bacteria traveled from the mouth to the brain. The researchers then discovered that the infected mouse brains had higher-than-normal levels of beta-amyloid, a protein closely linked to the development of AD.

Of course, lots more research — particularly on people — is needed to determine the interplay between gum disease and AD. In the meantime, you can do your part by maintaining good oral health. After all, gum disease has also been linked to serious health conditions like heart disease and diabetes.

Dental care helps keep up cognition. Your mom was right — you should brush your teeth twice a day. She probably knew you could get cavities or worse by neglecting your teeth. But she was also doing your brain a favor by making you brush and floss.

A study of Chinese American seniors found that those who reported having problems with their teeth were more likely to experience cognitive decline later in life. They were also more likely to have difficulties with episodic memory, which involves the ability to remember new information.

A lost tooth is no laughing matter. It can cause your jaw bone to shrink and your gums to become infected. Moreover, unrestored teeth can lead to cognitive impairment. How? Missing teeth make it difficult to chew. That can result in a loss of blood flow to the brain and mental decline.

Plaque happens: 4 reasons to do something about it

Did you know your mouth contains 700 types of bacteria? Before you dismiss the thought with an "ewww," you should know that untreated dental infections can wreak havoc on your body. Read on to see what you can do each day to cut the risks posed by harmful bacteria.

Plaque gums up the works for your heart and mind. Brushing and flossing your teeth daily may be the two easiest things you can do to help your heart and brain. Why? Because people with gum disease — a highly preventable condition — have twice the risk of heart attack or stroke. Fortunately, you may limit your risk of these life-threatening conditions by practicing good dental care each day.

Experts are still researching the connections between gum disease and cardiovascular problems. But they've found higher levels of an inflammation marker called C-reactive protein (CRP) in people with gum disease. Elevated levels of CRP appear to increase your risk of a heart attack. And inflammation can hamper blood and oxygen flow to the brain, increasing your chances of a stroke.

Dangerous intersection ahead at gum disease and diabetes. Inflammation is a key part of gum disease and diabetes. And scientists now believe these two conditions may actually fuel one another.

How? The bacteria that causes gum disease can migrate into your bloodstream. Naturally your body will put up a fight. That's good, but compounds produced by your immune reaction may raise your blood sugar. So if you have an ongoing problem like gum disease, then you could be setting yourself up with higher blood sugar levels over the long term. And that can lead to type 2 diabetes.

The reverse also seems to be true. People with unchecked diabetes run a higher risk of inflammation and gum disease. One possible reason? Diabetes can damage the blood vessels that supply nutrients to your gums. That can make it harder to fight infection.

Don't give arthritis a toothhold. A harmful bacteria called *Aggregatibacter actinomycetemcomitans (Aa)* has long been associated with the development of gum disease. And researchers now believe it can trigger an autoimmune response in people with rheumatoid arthritis (RA).

RA doesn't just cause painful and swollen joints. It can affect organs like your brain. In fact, many people with RA experience brain fog and have difficulty thinking. So what should you do? Keep your gums healthy by brushing gently twice a day, and get regular checkups and cleanings.

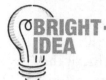

Seniors — sink your teeth into these tips for dental care

As you age, obstacles can crop up that make it hard to take care of your oral health. Arthritic hands don't always cooperate with fussy cleaning tools. Folks with mild cognitive impairment may forget parts of their daily dental routine. Don't let setbacks stop you from having a healthy mouth. You can adapt your routine and get back on track with a little creativity and almost no expense.

- If you forget to brush twice a day, post a note where you will see it regularly. Or set an alarm on your phone to remind you to floss daily.

- Floss failures? Long-handled flossers and floss threaders let you access all of your teeth easily.

- Get a better grip. Attach a piece of foam to make your toothbrush easier to hold.

- Dry mouth increases your tooth decay risk, so stay well hydrated with water.

- Still have dry mouth? Use a moisturizing spray regularly.

- Rinse and spit with water after a meal to dislodge bits of food and sugar.

- Forget squeezing the toothpaste. Lay the tube on the counter and press down. Or consider an automatic toothpaste dispenser.

- Stick to sugar-free gum.

- Visit your dentist. Cavities, gum disease, oral cancer, and dark teeth are not your friend. Your dentist is.

- Switch to low-acid food and drinks to protect your tooth enamel. Or be sure to sip water while eating or drinking something acidic.

- Learn to love low-fat foods. Lean meats can help rebuild your tooth enamel. And the calcium and protein in low-fat dairy can strengthen your teeth.

Dried fruit

The fruit that fosters your health in 5 flavorful ways

Plums, dates, apricots, figs — for millennia their sweetness has kept people coming back for more. But did you know drying them concentrates their antioxidants and extends their shelf life? Here are five other reasons dried fruit will have you coming back for more.

Munch on these for memory. Prunes, also known as dried plums, may seem like "old folk" food, but they could be key to a more youthful brain. They're high in boron, which is an amazing mineral that can help prevent a meltdown in mental functions like memory loss.

In a series of small studies, researchers found that low dietary boron in middle-aged and senior adults led to poorer performance on long- and short-term memory tasks compared to high boron intakes.

Not a fan of prunes? Raisins and dried apricots are also loaded with boron. Just stick to small servings. Dried fruits have a high concentration of fiber and fructose and could cause gas and bloating if you eat too much.

Key nutrients for thinking. In the same series of studies that looked at memory, researchers also found that low amounts of boron in the diet influenced other areas of cognitive function, such as attention and perception. But boron isn't the only nutrient in dried fruit involved in the brainpower business.

Vitamin K1 also seems to help mental function. Researchers had a group of seniors over age 75 in France complete a food survey, as well as tests that measured cognitive function and behavior problems linked to dementia, including self-control, mood problems, and loss of interest. And getting higher amounts of vitamin K1 was linked to better cognition and behavior.

Experts think vitamin K positively affects sphingolipids — parts of cells that play a role in brain function. Guess what? Prunes also happen to be high in vitamin K.

Dried fruits help motor skills. Grab a handful of raisins or dried apricots before your next game of catch with the grandkids. Why? They help keep your boron level up, which could support hand-eye coordination, including response time and manual dexterity.

Help yourself to healthier blood pressure. Anthocyanins in fruit may help reduce blood pressure. In several studies using powders from freeze-dried fruits including grapes and blueberries, participants saw decreases in systolic and diastolic blood pressure.

Raisins also show promise in lowering blood pressure, especially when compared to processed snacks. Good to know since research has linked high blood pressure to memory loss and a reduced ability to think quickly.

Bone up on dried fruit — your skeleton will thank you. Your bones are constantly being broken down and reformed in a process called bone remodeling. But with osteoporosis, you lose more than you regain, leaving your bones fragile. Amazingly, about eight dried plums a day helped improve bone mineral density in a clinical study of 160 postmenopausal women.

Why do experts say prunes are prime for supporting bone health? For one, they have a higher amount of vitamin K than many other fruits, which may protect bones by improving calcium balance. They're also brimming with boron, a nutrient that plays a role in bone development and regeneration.

No wonder researchers recommend dried plums for bone support in postmenopausal women. With powerful nutrients like that, young folks should be eating them, too. What's more, according to German researchers, osteoporosis is associated with a higher risk for dementia. As if you needed another reason to eat more dried fruit.

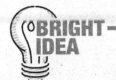

BRIGHT IDEA

DIY delights: Simple tips to dry your own fruit

Dried fruit isn't cheap. Not only that, fruit packaging may not tell you about added sulfites or sugars that quickly turn your healthy snack into a potential allergen or calorie bender. What can you do? Dry your own fruit.

Here's how to prepare clean, fresh fruit for drying.

- Core and slice when appropriate. Use a knife or food mandolin for thin, even slices.

- Some fruits like apples and pears change colors when cut because of exposure to air. Stop the browning by soaking the slices in an acidic solution for five minutes. Use a lemon juice and water mixture or soak them directly in orange, pineapple, or cranberry juice. Drain well.

- Leave berries whole. Put them in a colander and pour boiling water over them for four seconds. Spread them on a baking sheet and pat off excess moisture. Freeze one to two hours and they're ready to dry.

- Steam blanching fruit before drying also preserves color and freshness. Your steam time depends on the fruit but can range from three to eight minutes.

If you don't own a food dehydrator and would rather not buy one, you have other options for drying your fruit.

- Use an oven. Drying time usually runs six to 10 hours. Aim for 140 degrees. Prop the door open a couple of inches to allow air to circulate.

- Let your fruit bask in the warm sun, in dry temperatures over several days. You need the temperature to be above 86 degrees and the humidity below 60%.

- Make the most of your parked car's dash or back window over a couple of hot, sunny days when the inside temp reaches 100 degrees.

Rethink your cavity-fighting plan with raisins

If you've ever had a cavity, you were probably the victim of the bacteria known as *S. mutans*. Some folks would have you believe eating too many fruits caused your cavity, but the evidence just doesn't stack up. In fact, a fruit formerly held in high suspicion of dental high jinks — the raisin — has made headway in clearing its name with dentists. And it's ready to convince you, too.

In one study, scientists took 156 people and swabbed their teeth to get a cavity risk score. Then they gave half of the group a box of raisins to eat and half of the group nothing to eat. After 15 minutes, the researchers swabbed the participants' teeth again. The raisin group's cavity risk dropped, but the group that ate nothing did not see any change.

For all their healthy perks, dried fruits can quickly hike your sugar intake if you're not careful. Reach for a handful of prunes the next time you face a snack attack. These little powerhouses have the lowest sugar content per 100-gram serving compared to their cousins dried peaches and apricots.

The phytonutrients in these dried grapes seem to prevent bacteria from sticking to your teeth and stop the formation of plaque. And the more you can do to block bacteria buildup, the better. Scientists have found that bacteria in your mouth can move to your brain and release enzymes known to destroy nerve cells. That could lead to memory loss and Alzheimer's disease.

Eggs

Power up your plate with this brainy breakfast food

In the 1967 jailhouse flick "Cool Hand Luke," Paul Newman's character, Luke Jackson, brags that he can eat 50 hard-boiled eggs in one hour. The other prisoners bet against him, but Luke pulls through — finishing off all 50 in just under an hour. That's about 6 pounds of eggs. Fortunately, you won't need to eat that many eggs at a time to reap the brain benefits they offer.

What is it about eggs that make them so good for you? The choline. Never heard of it? That's OK. It's fairly new to the research game. In fact, it wasn't named an essential nutrient until 1998. Experts now know choline affects your liver, muscles, nervous system, heart, and of course, your brain. And they know your body needs choline to produce acetylcholine, a neurotransmitter — the body's chemical messenger — that helps regulate memory, mood, and intelligence.

Choline, an eggcellent nutrient for your brain. Choline research may have come late to the table — the nutrition table, that is — but experts are making up for lost time.

One recent study from Finland showed that the risk of dementia was 28% lower in men with the highest dietary intake of phosphatidyl-choline — a chemical partially made of choline — than men with the lowest intake. These men also did better on tests measuring memory and language abilities. Turns out choline is needed to synthesize DNA which is important for brain function.

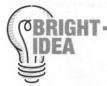

Chef's secret: How to boil the perfect egg

Scrambled, poached, fried, deviled. So many ways to prepare eggs. In fact, rumor has it, the number of pleats on chef hats was once a representation of how many ways the pro could serve up an egg. Some hats had as many as 100 pleats. But if you can't even boil an egg correctly, don't despair. Here are some do's and don'ts for preparing perfect boiled eggs, every time.

- Choose a pot that's right for the job. Don't pick a pot that's too small. Select one that allows the eggs to rest in a single layer and still have space to move around.

- Pick the proper eggs. Try not to use eggs that are too fresh. Instead, let them age in your fridge a week or two before you boil them to make them easier to peel.

- Don't start with boiling water. Place your eggs in the pot and cover them with about an inch of cool water.

- Cook the eggs for the right amount of time. Bring the water to a boil, take the pot off the heat and cover it. For soft-boiled eggs, let it sit four to six minutes. For hard-boiled eggs, rest it eight to 12 minutes.

- Follow with an ice bath so your eggs won't continue to cook. Drain off the water and carefully move your eggs to a bowl containing ice and water. Soak until the eggs are cool.

How choline may lower the risk for Alzheimer's disease (AD).
A new study out of Arizona State University found that supplementing with choline improved memory in the offspring of mice bred to display AD-like symptoms. The researchers explored two ways choline may protect against the memory-stealing disease.

- Choline reduces unhealthy levels of a protein-building amino acid called homocysteine that can contribute to the development of amyloid plaques, a well-known sign of Alzheimer's disease. In fact, high levels of homocysteine actually double the risk of developing AD. But choline changes dangerous homocysteine into the helpful chemical methionine, a protein-building essential amino acid.

> Can't decide if an egg is fresh? Use the float test. Place your egg in a bowl of water. If the egg sinks, it's fresh. It will stand on one end or float if it's old. To determine if it's safe to eat, crack or peel it and check for an off-odor or unusual appearance.

- Choline also tames microglia — cells that act as an immune defense for the brain and spinal cord but can cause brain inflammation and even neuronal death when they become overactive. Choline reduces the activation of microglia which then helps protect the brain from AD.

How much choline do you need? Men should get 550 milligrams (mg) of choline per day, while women should strive for 425 mg per day. A hard-boiled egg will get you part of the way there with its generous 147 mg of choline.

A trio of perks from one savory source

So you think you're pretty good at multitasking — doing several things at once. For example, you can listen to the radio and talk on the phone while you balance your checkbook. Beware. Researchers say multitasking can actually knock your productivity by up to 40%.

But where food's concerned, eggs are the ultimate multitasker. Besides keeping your brain operating on the sunny side, eggs boost your health in three ways you're probably not expecting. What a pip!

Egg on your weight loss. Scientists have discovered that having extra pounds around the middle is linked with brain shrinkage. How can eggs help you lose weight?

Researchers conducted an eight-week study of 152 overweight or obese — but otherwise healthy — men and women between the ages of 25 and 60 who either followed a reduced-calorie diet or stuck with their regular eating habits. All participants were assigned to eat either an egg breakfast consisting of two scrambled eggs, toast, and jelly, or a bagel breakfast made up of a bagel, cream cheese, and yogurt for at least five days per week.

At the end of the study, the dieters eating eggs instead of bagels showed a 65% greater weight loss, a 34% greater drop in waist measurement, and a 16% greater reduction in body fat percentage. The researchers also discovered that if the participants weren't following a diet, the egg plan did not help them lose weight.

> Ahoy, matey! Pirate lore says chickens were kept on board ships to provide eggs for the crew. Cackle fruit, they called them. Pirates probably weren't concerned about the myth connecting cholesterol to eggs. And you may not need to worry, either. Today's researchers think an egg a day may not increase your risk of heart disease. Shiver me timbers!

Previous studies have demonstrated the satisfying effects of eggs, a high-protein meal, compared to a high-carbohydrate breakfast like the bagel breakfast. You feel full, longer.

See clearly with this breakfast eye-opener. All eyes are on one study that found people with age-related macular degeneration (AMD) were 20% more likely to develop dementia compared with people who didn't have AMD.

This eye disease happens when part of your eye's retina — called the macula — is damaged. Your side vision will seem fine, but you lose your central vision. For example, pretend you're looking at a clock with hands. You may see all the numbers around the edge, but not the hands in the center. That's what AMD is like.

Making eggs a part of your diet may help you avoid AMD. Eggs contain lutein and zeaxanthin, two nutrients that block blue light from reaching the retina which may lower the risk of light-induced oxidative damage linked to AMD.

Researchers recently found that folks who ate two to four eggs each week reduced their risk of developing wet AMD by 62% compared to those who ate one or fewer. Wet AMD happens when abnormal blood vessels leak fluid or blood into the macula and is a leading cause of irreversible blindness.

Start your day with better sugar control. The dangers of out-of-control glucose are well known. Just one instance of high blood sugar can be harmful to the brain, resulting in problems with memory and attention. Researchers say breakfast is often the meal that causes the biggest sugar spike for folks with type 2 diabetes. Eggs can help with that.

In a two-day study, participants ate an omelet for breakfast one day, and ate oatmeal and fruit on another. Dinner and lunch were identical on both days.

The study found that beginning the day with a very low-carb, high-fat breakfast — the omelet — stopped the blood sugar spike. And this had enough of an effect to help stabilize participants' glucose readings for the next 24 hours.

Fermented foods

Take control of your gut to protect your brain

Your brain is like the captain of a ship — the overseer and commander of operations. But if things aren't working properly below deck — in your belly — your brain may suffer the consequences. In fact, a healthy gut could be the key to preventing one of Americans' most feared diseases. That's why eating fermented foods, which keep your intestinal track strong and healthy, may reduce your chances of developing Alzheimer's disease. Plus, these tangy victuals may ease anxiety levels.

Fermentation occurs when microbes convert the sugars in a food into lactic acid. It's what turns cabbage into sauerkraut and cucumbers into pickles. Not only does the process preserve the food, it promotes the growth of healthy bacteria that keep your gastrointestinal tract in tiptop condition.

Probiotics help defend against Alzheimer's disease. Experts believe Alzheimer's disease (AD) develops when beta-amyloid plaques build up in your brain. But your gut may play more of a role than you expect. That's because your central nervous system and gastrointestinal tract are connected through a communication system called the gut-brain axis. In fact, the link is so strong that harmful bacteria in your gut may increase your risk of Alzheimer's disease. How? By releasing amyloid proteins that eventually accumulate in your brain.

Only a few studies have reported on the impact fermented foods might have on cognitive function. But some researchers have found that healthy diets that include high amounts of probiotics — the beneficial bacteria and yeasts found in fermented foods — reduce the risk of developing AD.

It also appears that probiotics may delay cognitive decline. A study published in *Frontiers in Aging Neuroscience* found that seniors with AD who drank a little less than a cup of probiotic milk daily for 12 weeks showed significant improvements on cognitive tests compared with a control group that drank regular milk.

Scientists aren't really sure why probiotics seem to help cognitive function. But they say it may be due to probiotics' ability to rebalance the levels of good and bad bacteria in your gut. Probiotics also may help fight oxidative stress and insulin resistance, two conditions linked to AD.

Calm anxiety symptoms from the belly on up. Researchers published in *General Psychiatry* say taking probiotic supplements may brighten your mood. They reviewed 14 studies of people who used probiotics to regulate their intestinal bacteria and found that more than a third of the participants reported reduced anxiety symptoms, including feeling less irritable and restless.

Among these studies, one commonly used probiotic was *Lactobacillus*. You may find one species of this helpful healer, called *L. acidophilus*, in your favorite yogurt. You can also get your fill with other fermented foods like cheese, tempeh, miso, and sauerkraut.

When it comes to fermented foods, moderation and reading the label are key. Sure, they contain helpful probiotics that may improve blood pressure and blood sugar. But other ingredients can cancel out the benefits. Sodium-rich foods like kimchi and pickles can raise your blood pressure. And some yogurts have a boatload of added sugar.

BRIGHT IDEA

6 steps to fabulous fermented foods

Want to improve your produce's shelf life and your health? Fermentation is the way to go. People have been perfecting this art for thousands of years. With the heavy lifting already done, you can get started with just six simple steps.

- Pick out your produce. Pesticides kill good bacteria, so go organic. Popular veggie choices include cucumbers, cabbage, and green beans. Thoroughly wash them, and then chop them into strips or chunks.

- Get a good container. Don't spend big bucks on fancy fermentation jars. Use Mason jars that have been washed and air-dried instead.

- Decide if you will use salt or a starter culture — a strong bacterial strain you can buy online or at health stores — to kick off the fermentation process.

- Pour your veggies, seasoning, and filtered water into your mason jar. Adding salt or a starter is key to killing bad microbes and promoting good bacteria. Three tablespoons of salt per 5 pounds of veggies is typical. But if you're on a low-sodium diet, add just enough salt to taste and a starter. Make sure all of your produce is completely covered in the brine.

- Screw on your Mason jar's lid until it's lightly snug. You want to allow carbon dioxide to escape.

- Store your jar in a dark, cool place. Fermentation time can vary dramatically, so taste periodically until your fermented veggies reach your preferred level of tartness. At that point, it's time for storage in the fridge.

Pick me: Fermented fare helps heart to brain

It's hard to believe fermentation was probably an accidental discovery. But you can thank your ancestors for stumbling across this naturally healthy method of preserving food. After all, fermented foods have helped heal bodies for over 6,000 years.

Fermented dairy is a natural heart remedy. Lift your glass and toast your Scandinavian friends with a rousing "Skål" next time you get a hankering for fermented milk. You might even ask for seconds after learning that this traditional Northern European drink may lower your risk of having a heart attack. Yogurt and cheese are two other fermented dairy products that may benefit your cardiovascular health. That's because fermented dairy may help reduce inflammation more than unfermented dairy.

So heap some of these foods onto your plate when your stomach is rumbling. Researchers who followed nearly 2,000 middle-aged men over 20 years found that those who ate the most fermented dairy — cheese, yogurt, kefir, and fermented milk — had a 27% lower risk of having a heart attack, chest pain, or cardiac arrest due to coronary heart disease. None of the men had heart disease at the beginning of the study.

Additional research suggests that fermented dairy can also reduce your blood pressure and lower your risk of stroke. That's important because high blood pressure can cause the arteries that supply blood to your brain to burst or get blocked, causing a stroke. Depending on the part of your brain that is affected, a stroke can damage your memory, motor skills, speech, behavior, and thought processes.

Eat to lose weight with yogurt and kimchi. Your brain is vulnerable to conditions like diabetes, high blood pressure, and heart disease. All of which can arise from obesity. But filling up on probiotics — the live bacteria found in fermented foods — may protect against these dangers by helping you shed unwanted pounds.

A study of more than 38,800 adults found that those who took probiotics — either by eating yogurt or taking supplements — were 17% less likely to be obese. What's more, they were 21% less likely to have high blood pressure. Not a fan of yogurt? Kimchi is another fermented food linked with anti-obesity and anti-hypertension properties.

Your bowel benefits from probiotics. Irritable bowel syndrome (IBS) is a chronic condition that affects the large intestine and can cause abdominal pain, diarrhea, and constipation. Unfortunately, medication doesn't always adequately treat all of the symptoms. But probiotics may provide relief.

That's according to researchers who reviewed nine studies on people with IBS. They found that compared with control groups, the people who took probiotics benefited from reduced abdominal pain, bloating, and gas after just four to eight weeks of treatment. In addition, their overall quality of life improved. Researchers think probiotics help by regulating the balance of good and bad bacteria in your intestines and aiding your immune system.

Improving your gut health can help clear up your mind, too. That's because the symptoms of IBS have been linked to brain fog, a condition that makes it difficult to concentrate and remember things.

Combat inflammation with friendly bacteria. Dietary changes, infection, and antibiotics can wreak havoc on the trillions of bacteria in your gut. That can throw off your intestinal immune system's ability to function properly and lead to the development of inflammatory bowel disease.

Also called IBD, this disorder is more than a little tummy trouble. The chronic inflammation can damage your gastrointestinal tract

> Captain James Cook had some special cargo aboard his ship when he and his sailors left England for the South Pacific in 1768. Can't guess what it was? Nearly 8,000 pounds of fermented cabbage. Turns out the live lactic bacteria in sauerkraut promotes the absorption of vitamin C, a key way to fend off scurvy.

and even affect your brain. A study of adults with Crohn's disease — one of the two forms of IBD — found that they had slower response times on cognitive tests than people without the disease. The researchers believe bowel inflammation can cause increased inflammatory activity in the brain, resulting in cloudy thinking.

Probiotics often contain lactic acid-producing bacteria that can improve the health of your intestinal tract. And research suggests that one in particular, called *Lactobacilli*, can ease IBD symptoms. That's because this type of bacteria appears to help move food through your digestive system and relieve IBD-related constipation.

Decipher supplement labels with ease

Supplements aren't a replacement for a healthy lifestyle, but they can give you a probiotic bonus. Just check with your doctor before taking them because they may interact with your medications. Here's how to easily understand their complicated labels.

- Name. Look for the genus, species, and strain of bacteria. You need all three because health benefits can vary between strains.

- Recommended use. This tells you how you may benefit from the product.

- Testing. Check for third-party testing. A seal from USP, ConsumerLab, or NSF provides confirmation.

- Dose. This is how much you need to get the advertised benefits.

- Colony Forming Units (CFU). Avoid products with CFU "at time of manufacture" because the amount of live culture can decline over time.

- Expiration date. This tells you how long the probiotic bacteria will deliver claimed benefits.

- Proper storage. Look for storage information to ensure quality and safety.

Fiber

Diamond in the roughage: Eat your way to better brain health

Do you ever find yourself weighing a decision your gut and brain can't agree on? Maybe it's simple — like what's for dinner. Your gut calls for unhealthy carbs, but your brain says think twice. If those carbs come from fiber-rich whole grains, fruits, and vegetables, however, feel free to pull up to the table and chow down. Why? Fiber-rich foods can keep both your brain and gut healthy.

Fiber cleans out inflammation. A type of immune cell in your brain — called microglia — tends to become overactive and inflamed as you get older. It's one of the reasons your memories may fade and other mental functions may deteriorate with age.

Your gut can also get inflamed, in part because the good and bad bacteria living there develop an imbalance. Moreover, older folks have lower amounts of bacteria that make sodium butyrate, a short-chain fatty acid that supports digestive health and helps control inflammation.

But new research suggests that eating a high-fiber diet may spark a chemical response that solves these problems. Scientists who fed aging mice either a high- or low-fiber diet over four weeks found that those on the high-fiber diet had increased levels of sodium butyrate at the end of the study. The mice on the high-fiber diet also had less inflammation in their intestinal tract and microglial cells.

Of course, the results need to be translated to humans. But if they hold true, it's just one more reason to make sure you get enough fiber from fruits, vegetables, beans and whole grains.

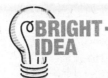

Tips for bridging the fiber gap

It fights heart disease, normalizes blood sugar, eases digestion, stimulates weight loss, even improves your mood. But a national survey shows as few as 5% of Americans eat enough of this healing ingredient in their food. Discover easy, inexpensive, delicious ways to get more fiber.

Women over age 50 need at least 21 grams of fiber a day. Men in the same age bracket need at least 30 grams a day. While processed foods with added fiber will help you meet those goals, they rarely contain the vitamins, minerals, and other nutrients you'll find in natural, high-fiber foods like fruits, vegetables, and whole grains.

Good news, though. You can make simple swaps and easy additions to your diet to get all the fiber you need.

- Swap white flour for whole-grain flour.

- Add beans to your soup or salad instead of meat.

- Drop a scoop of granola and dried fruit into your yogurt.

- Trade low-fiber cereals for ones with whole grains listed as the first ingredient.

- Mix a teaspoon of unsweetened cocoa powder into your coffee for an extra half gram of fiber. But don't forget that cocoa powder also has caffeine.

- Sneak a tablespoon of unsweetened cocoa into your next batch of chili.

- Sprinkle nutritional yeast into your soups and whole-wheat pasta. Or add it to popcorn in place of butter and salt.

- Blend leafy greens with berries, a banana, lemon juice, and ice water for a refreshing green smoothie.

Happy guts make happier lives.
Did you know that intestinal
bacteria "talk" with your brain via
the hormone cortisol? But that's
not all these microbes are good
for. Gut bacteria make 90% of
the mood-boosting chemical
serotonin in your body. And what
helps them thrive? Prebiotics —
types of fiber that feed the friendly
bacteria in your intestinal tract.

Put down that plain bagel
and reach for oatmeal.
Studies show that people
with colorectal cancer who
ate a high-fiber diet had a
significantly lower risk of
dying from the disease than
those who ate a low-fiber
diet. The type of roughage
that helped? Whole grains
and cereal fiber.

In turn, good bacteria change your gut for the better — meaning
you could experience healthier digestion, improved memory, and
an elevated mood. After all, nobody wants to feel blue — and
depression has been linked to forgetfulness and confusion.

Fit more fiber into your diet to keep your gut and your mind on
the sunny side of life. These tasty foods are packed with prebiotics.

- chicory, Jerusalem artichokes, garlic, and leeks

- bananas, grapefruit, apples, and watermelon

- chickpeas, lentils, and soybeans

Bulk up to stay fit as a fiddle

What's the secret to a long life? Stay healthy, right? That's obvious,
but researchers conducting a study were surprised to find that seniors
who ate the most fiber were more likely to live longer. That's because
they were less likely to suffer from debilitating health problems like
cancer and dementia. Maybe it's time to take a fiber inventory in
your pantry.

Kick cholesterol to the curb. Long-term studies suggest that a
diet high in soluble fiber — the kind of fiber that absorbs water
and turns to gel during digestion — can protect you from heart
disease because it lowers cholesterol.

How does it work? Soluble fiber binds to cholesterol in your small intestine. So instead of entering your bloodstream and migrating to your arteries, the cholesterol gets eliminated from your body. That's important because clear arteries keep oxygen-rich blood flowing to your brain.

Waist, not! Your fiber opportunity. Obesity opens the door to conditions like diabetes, high blood pressure, and heart disease that can negatively affect your brain. But fiber is an ally in weight loss efforts.

A review of dozens of studies found that adults who added soluble fiber to their regular diets lost more weight than those who didn't. They also saw greater reductions in their body mass index and size of their waists. Overweight people and those with diabetes or metabolic syndrome benefited the most.

This type of fiber helps you lose weight because it slows digestion, making you feel full longer.

Defend yourself against high blood sugar. Scientists have found potential connections between problems with how the brain processes glucose and Alzheimer's disease. Diabetes also poses risks to your overall health, so it's best to do everything possible to prevent it.

Need to lower your blood sugar? A 12-week study of people with type 2 diabetes found that those who ate a high-fiber diet had greater reductions in their average fasting glucose levels than a control group on a standard diet. They also lost more weight.

The researchers say the high-fiber diet promoted the growth of gut bacteria that produced short-chain fatty acids. The acids made the intestinal tracts of the fiber-eating participants less hospitable to harmful bacteria. The result? The amount of bad bacteria in their guts dropped.

> Your gut is absolutely amazing. It has 100 million neurons that form an independent nervous system. That's why your intestinal tract is often referred to as a "second brain." To top it off, the trillions of microbes in your gut produce chemicals that your brain uses to regulate your body.

The acids also led to increases in insulin production and better glucose control, the scientists say.

Nutrition labels: 2 fiber facts you must know

Not every grain helps your digestive tract — so look for the "100% whole grain" label before you buy a product. And not every carbohydrate contains fiber. Take a good look at nutrition labels to see what you're really eating.

What is fiber? The FDA defines fiber as a non-digestible carbohydrate found in plants or, if not natural, one that is added and has proven health benefits.

What's included on a label? Manufacturers can freely list naturally occurring fiber — cereal bran, vegetables, and whole grains, for example — on their Nutrition and Supplement Facts labels.

They can also include some artificial fibers that the FDA has vetted for health benefits such as the ability to lower blood sugar or relieve constipation. Psyllium husk, pectin, and cellulose are some of the added fibers that can be included on nutrition labels.

Fish

Catch of the day keeps your brain on an even keel

If one food could lower your risk of developing Alzheimer's disease (AD), stroke, and heart disease, wouldn't you be stockpiling it in your fridge? What if the nutrients in this same food could protect you from arthritis, cataracts, weak bones, poor digestion, and even some cancers? Believe it or not, you can get this superfood at any supermarket.

Sound a little fishy? It is! Here's how to reel in the nutrients you need to help you live longer and keep your brain sharp.

This nutrient-packed delight fights forgetfulness. It's no fish tale. Researchers discovered that people who ate baked or broiled fish — sorry, no fried fish here — just once a week had a lower chance of developing AD.

The study looked at a group of 260 men and women who didn't have AD or serious memory problems. Those who ate fish at least once a week had larger gray matter volume in areas of the brain responsible for memory and cognition compared to those who ate fish less often. That's good news because greater brain volume may signal that memory and thinking functions are being maintained. Brain shrinkage, on the other hand, has been linked to AD.

"Consuming baked or broiled fish promotes stronger neurons in the brain's gray matter by making them larger and healthier," said Dr. Cyrus Raji of the University of Pittsburgh. "This simple lifestyle choice increases the brain's resistance to Alzheimer's disease and lowers risk for the disorder."

Catch a wave of protection for your brain. Two weekly servings of fish can reduce your risk of stroke, say researchers at Harvard Medical School.

They found that women who ate 4 ounces of fish, about the size of a deck of cards, two to four times a week cut their risk of stroke caused by blood clots — called thrombotic strokes — by about 50%. That's compared to women who ate fish less than once a month.

It's the omega-3 fatty acids in dark, oily fish like salmon, mackerel, and sardines that net you such swell results. These healthy fats can help reduce the stickiness of platelets, the cells that help form blood clots. And since clots cause 80% of strokes, keeping your blood vessels clot-free can ward off your stroke risk.

> Fish sauce is typically made of anchovies and salt aged in barrels for six months or longer. The salt takes out the moisture and preserves the anchovies, allowing them to ferment which gives the sauce its unique taste. Enjoy it in marinades, soups, or stir-fries. But remember, a little sprinkle goes a long way.

Angling to improve your memory? Then you'll like this fish story. A team of researchers found that eating a meal of foods containing omega-3 fatty acids at least once a week might protect older adults against age-related memory loss and thinking problems.

The five-year study followed 915 participants who were an average of 81 years old. They were divided into two groups — those who ate at least one seafood meal per week, and those who ate less than one seafood meal per week.

The people who ate more seafood had lower rates of decline in memory of verbal information. They also had slower rates of decline on a test that measured their ability to quickly compare letters, objects, and patterns.

"This study helps show that while cognitive abilities naturally decline as part of the normal aging process, there is something that we can do to mitigate this process," says Martha Clare Morris, Sc.D., senior author of the paper.

Here's a lifesaver for your heart. Three cheers for those omega-3 fatty acids. Experts think omega-3s can reduce inflammation throughout your body — the kind of inflammation that could damage your blood vessels, raising your risk for heart disease.

What else can omega-3 fatty acids do? They may decrease your triglycerides, a kind of fat found in your blood that can contribute to hardening of the arteries. Omega-3s also help lower your blood pressure and reduce blood clotting. That's why the American Heart Association recommends two servings of fish a week to support your ticker.

So if you're looking for a brain saver and a heart helper all in one tasty dish, try fish. You'll be hooked in no time.

Food for thought: Balance your gut to protect your brain

When your body detects invaders — like bacteria, viruses, and other organisms that can cause infections — it launches an army of white blood cells to clear them out. That's the healing process. Inflammation plays an important role in that process, but sometimes it can go too far and damage your healthy cells, which can lead to memory and thinking problems.

Smoking, stress, and alcohol are just a few of the causes of inflammation gone amuck. Another, often overlooked cause? An imbalance in your gut's microbiome.

Your gut — the highway to better health. You are mostly microbes. Over 100 trillion of them. The majority live in harmony, for the most part, in your gut — especially in the large intestine. Amazingly, this community of microbes — known as your microbiome — may weigh as much as 5 pounds.

The microbiome's jobs include digesting food, regulating your immune system, and producing vitamins like thiamine, riboflavin, and vitamin K. But when the microbes get out of whack through a change in your diet, poor dental hygiene, or new meds like antibiotics, all kinds of problems could crop up — including brain woes. Seems weird, doesn't it? But it's true. Your gut and your brain are connected.

In fact, a recent study revealed that the balance of gut microbes in folks with dementia and those without dementia are different. And this led the researchers to suggest that your microbiome has an effect on brain health, including the development of dementia. Experts think emotions and mood could be affected by your microbiome, too.

And that's not all. Want to prevent chronic illnesses like diabetes, heart disease, and high blood pressure? Even reduce belly fat? Researchers are hopeful that improving the gut microbiome could be the focus of future treatments.

Get control of your gut's balancing act. Since your diet shapes your microbiome, what should you eat to keep it healthy? Experts say it may be a good idea to load up on omega-3s. They discovered that getting more of these fatty acids was linked to improved microbiome diversity in middle-aged and senior women. And that's good because having a more diverse microbiome is tied to lower inflammation, among other health benefits.

What's a great source of these fatty acids? Fish, of course. Studies have connected health benefits to intakes that average out between 250 and 500 milligrams (mg) of omega-3 fatty acids a day. You'll get a boatload of the nutrient when you dig into these fish.

- 3-ounce serving of farmed salmon (1,921 mg)
- 3-ounce serving of herring (1,885 mg)
- 3-ounce serving of mackerel (1,209 mg)
- 3.75-ounce can of sardines (1,362 mg)
- 2-ounce can of anchovies (951 mg)

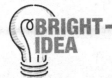

BRIGHT IDEA

Farmed vs. wild — straight facts to find what floats your boat

You've heard of aquatics, aqualungs, and aquarium. Even Aquaman. That "aqua" at the front gives away the meaning of the words, so you know they all have to do with water. But how about aquaculture? You might be surprised to learn it's the business of producing healthy omega-3 fatty acids for your dinner table.

According to the National Oceanic and Atmospheric Administration (NOAA), aquaculture is the breeding and harvesting of fish, shellfish, and algae. Fish farming, you might say. Aquaculture is generally done in net pens in the water, in tanks on land, or in ponds or other man-made systems.

So which is best? Fish caught in the wild or fish that is farmed using aquaculture? Here's your chance to compare them fin to fin, and pick the one that floats your boat.

- Nutrition. Farmed salmon has more omega-3s than wild-caught salmon, but it also has more calories and saturated fat. Wild salmon is higher in potassium, zinc, and iron.

- Price. Wild salmon is often more expensive than farmed. Consider frozen or canned wild-caught salmon as cheaper alternatives.

Does it matter where your seafood comes from? You bet. Some overseas sources of both wild-caught and farm-raised fish could be higher in contaminants like mercury. Antibiotic use in farm-raised fish is common, too. To find out where your fish is from, check the Country of Origin Labeling (COOL) on the package, now required on all seafood sold in the U.S.

Gardening

Everything's coming up roses: Sow the seeds of a healthy mind

Perennials are flowers that keep coming back, season after season. Something you may relate to as you blossom in your senior years. In fact, some people use the word "perennials" to describe baby boomers who want to stay active and feel their best as they age. Planting your favorite long-lasting flower is one way to do just that.

Ward off Alzheimer's disease with gardening. The children's book *Miss Rumphius* is inspired by the real story of Hilda Hamlin. She's known for scattering lupine seeds along the coast of Maine, a hobby that earned her the nickname "Lupine Lady." Fortunately, you don't have to trek so far to benefit from gardening.

The physical activity you get in your own backyard will do. Researchers studied five years of data on almost 900 adults who were age 65 or older. They found that those who burned the most calories through exercise — gardening, dancing, and walking, for example — had larger brain volumes in areas responsible for memory and cognition. They also had a reduced risk of developing Alzheimer's disease.

Don't feel up to a strenuous workout? No worries. Research suggests that even light exercise can help promote the growth of nerve cells in your brain. A study published in the *International Journal of Environmental Research and Public Health* found that 20 minutes of low- to moderate-intensity work in your garden is all you need.

Got a flower bed? Lay stress and fatigue to rest. If you feel overwhelmed, try communing with nature for instant relief.

Reconnecting with the great outdoors can reduce blood pressure and muscle tension — two symptoms of stress. Nurturing plants may help you get to the root of the problem.

Gardening helps reduce stress and fatigue, according to researchers. Scientists in England found that tending a community garden for just 30 minutes can bestow these benefits. And they don't fade if you repeat this routine just once a week.

A green thumb raises happiness levels. Did you know that gardening can improve your mood? A study of 370 people in Minnesota found that, across the study's population, the level of happiness reported while gardening at home was similar to what people reported during activities like biking, walking, or dining out. In fact, gardening was near the top of the activity list in terms of the happiness it gave people.

How much time did the gardeners commit to their hobby? About 90 minutes a week.

And the type of garden that appeared to offer the most satisfaction? Vegetable gardens. That's because producing your own food offers a trifecta of health benefits — fresh food, physical activity, and emotional well-being.

> Spending time outdoors in your garden is a terrific way to soak up rays. Your skin converts the ultraviolet light from the sun into vitamin D. Your body makes less of this key nutrient as you age, but gardening for just one hour a week can help make sure you get enough.

Backyard paradises help your heart and waist

The Secret Garden is a beloved children's novel by British American author Frances Hodgson Burnett. A tale of self-healing, the main characters cultivate newfound health and friendship through their shared love of bringing an abandoned garden back to life. Although the story is fictional, it's a fact that tending outdoor plants can help keep heart disease at bay and your weight in check.

Reap better heart health with your harvest. Heart disease is the leading cause of death in the U.S. But according to researchers, any kind of physical activity can help reduce your risk for coronary heart disease and cardiovascular disease.

A five-year study of 5,900 older women suggests that even light exercise — gardening or going for a stroll, for example — has tremendous benefits. And the more of it you get, the better.

- Women in the study who had the highest level of light physical activity — a little more than 5 1/2 hours a day — had a 42% lower risk of heart attack and coronary death than women who got around four hours or less.

- The most active women in this study also had a 22% lower risk of stroke and heart failure.

And when you help your heart, you help your brain. That's because heart attacks and strokes can restrict the flow of oxygen-rich blood to your brain.

This gym alternative keeps your waist trim. Have you ever felt so overwhelmed at the gym that you didn't want to go back? If so, gardening may be the perfect choice for you. It's easy to weave into your daily routine and is a good way to transition into a more active lifestyle.

When you garden, you get a workout all over. And that helps you control your weight. A study in the *American Journal of Public Health* found that people who worked in their community garden had a significantly lower body mass index than their neighbors who didn't.

That may not come as a surprise since gardening is an excellent way to burn calories. Expect to use up 200 to 400 calories every hour you're gardening. And while you're outdoors, bask in the new way you've helped your brain. Conditions arising from obesity, including diabetes and high blood pressure, can damage your blood vessels and lead to cognitive decline.

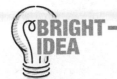

Got arthritis? These tips will tame the pain

Gardening is a great way to maintain your strength, joint flexibility, and range of motion. But sometimes people with arthritis find it difficult to bend, stoop, and dig. If that sounds like you, consider these tips to make your gardening life easier.

- Warm up before gardening and cool down afterward with a few light stretches. You'll reduce joint inflammation. Making circles with your arms and ankles is a good option.

- Use raised planters to minimize bending and putting strain on your back, knees, shoulders, and arms.

- Save energy by planting your garden close to a water source and storing your tools nearby.

- Grow low-maintenance herbs like basil, chives, cilantro, and dill.

- Weed when the ground is still wet from rain. The weeds are easier to pull.

- Choose ergonomic tools that minimize effort and discomfort. For hand tools, look for handles that keep your wrist straight. Pick long-handled tools that will help avoid back and hip strain caused by bending.

- Avoid kneeling whenever possible. If you have to kneel, get down on one knee and use a pad.

- When picking up objects, bend and then use your leg muscles to straighten up. Keep your back as straight as possible and hold the object close to your body.

- Switch tasks at least every 20 minutes to work different muscle groups. You'll minimize repetitive stress on your spine, joints, and muscles.

- Take breaks to stretch and rehydrate.

Ginseng

Think and see better: Ginseng gets to the root of what ails you

Folklore has it that medicinal plants look like the part of the body they help treat. Ginseng is a plant whose mature root resembles the human body. That's one reason people have thought of it as a cure-all for over 2,000 years. These days, the most-studied way to experience the wonder of this herb is through supplements that boast benefits for a wide range of conditions.

Limit the effects of Alzheimer's disease (AD). People who suffer from AD often have trouble with memory, language, and thinking skills. Given that ginseng is known to affect the nervous system — which plays a role in all three — researchers tested Korean red ginseng (KRG) on cognitive function in people with AD.

They chose 61 people who were already taking dementia medication and divided them into three groups. Each day participants took 4.5 grams of KRG, 9 grams of KRG, or a placebo. Before and after the 12-week study, they took tests that measured cognitive and functional performance related to AD. The findings? Those taking the highest dose of KRG scored better compared to the control group.

Ginseng helps calm anxiety and stress. Compared to other medicinal plants, ginseng has an impressive ability to regulate stress — a major cause of depression.

Stress provokes a network of reactions in your body.

- It triggers the HPA axis — the communication between the hypothalamus in your brain, its neighboring pituitary gland,

and your adrenal gland just above your kidneys. As a result, your body produces the hormone cortisol to handle the stress. But too much cortisol can affect brain function in areas associated with depression.

• Stress also lowers levels of a protein called brain-derived neurotrophic factor (BDNF) which may cripple your brain's ability to protect itself against depression.

In animal studies, the biologically active parts of ginseng — called ginsenosides — helped fight stress and depression by regulating the HPA axis and increasing BDNF.

Keep your vision sharp. Poor vision can limit your ability to participate in activities that stimulate your brain. But ginsenosides may be helpful in the fight against vision-stealing diseases.

• One study suggests KRG extract may slow the development of age-related macular degeneration.

• Another study shows that people with glaucoma had fewer dry eye symptoms after taking 3 grams a day of a KRG supplement for eight weeks.

• Animal and test tube studies point to ginseng as a possible remedy to prevent cataracts and damage to cells inside the eye.

No herbal supplement or preparation is perfect. Despite ginseng's track record of health benefits, occasionally people experience side effects like insomnia, nervousness, skin reactions, or digestive problems. Ask your doctor before starting a ginseng supplement because it may interact with certain medications like warfarin, aspirin, heparin, and antidepressants.

An herb for all occasions backs your brain in unexpected ways

One of the first successful trading expeditions the newly formed United States sent to China carried more than 30 tons of the all-healing herb American ginseng. They returned with a 25% profit.

What makes ginseng so desirable? It could lessen stress and improve memory. The Chinese merchants knew this popular remedy from their own Asian varieties. With its brain benefits revealed to the West at last, ginseng has made quite the splash in both markets. Here are three more ways this herb may be kind to your mind.

Boast better blood sugar. High blood sugar can damage your blood vessels, which could result in poor blood circulation to your brain. That can make it difficult to think.

Fortunately, a review of 16 trials showed ginseng lowered the fasting blood glucose in people with and without diabetes compared to control groups.

But here's some news. Fermented red ginseng may be better at blood sugar control. The fermentation process seems to make its ginsenosides easier for your body to absorb. Case in point — participants in a clinical trial took 2.7 grams of fermented red ginseng (FRG) a day or placebo for four weeks. As a result, the FRG group had lower blood glucose levels and higher insulin levels following a meal, signaling an improvement in the glucose-stimulated insulin response.

Fettered by fatigue? Ginseng might help. People suffering from chronic fatigue are often stressed and sleep poorly, which only makes memory problems worse. But researchers think ginseng might offer some relief.

They fed mice amino acids called ginseng oligopeptides (GOP) — taken from Asian ginseng — and gave a control group distilled water for 30 days. The GOP mice had more energy and outlasted the control group in a swimming test.

Are you tired from lack of sleep? One small study suggests red ginseng extract (RGE) may improve sleep quality. Healthy volunteers took 1,500 milligrams of RGE three times a day for a week and spent more time asleep while in bed than before taking ginseng.

Ginseng may have a hearty effect on your ticker. High blood pressure is a leading cause of strokes. And no wonder. It can cause structural changes in your heart and arteries as they adapt to the increased pressure.

One study of animals with high blood pressure showed that two ginsenosides from ginseng reduced negative changes in heart structure and function, even without lowering blood pressure. That's why researchers suggest ginseng compounds may protect the heart and blood vessels.

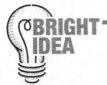

BRIGHT IDEA

Dig up the truth about choosing a supplement

What do folks do with ginseng after harvesters — known as sengers — do the dirty work of digging up the root? Some stew it in soups, make teas, or serve it up in stir-fry. You can even find it in soaps, eye masks, and energy drinks. More than ever, people look for it as a supplement in liquid, powder, or capsule forms.

But as more and more products flood the market, finding the right one can be tricky. Here's how to root through your options.

Pay close attention to the type of ginseng in your supplement. Researchers tend to use two basic varieties known as Asian or Korean ginseng (*Panax ginseng*) and American ginseng (*Panax quinquefolius*). Both varieties can be processed in three ways that change the levels of different ginsenosides.

- Red ginseng has been steamed and dried.

- White ginseng has been dried and peeled.

- Black ginseng has been dried and steamed more than once.

Siberian ginseng carries the name, but it doesn't have the helpful ginsenosides.

Choose wisely — not all supplements are equal. Ginseng supplements are generally considered safe, but lab tests have shown that some products don't contain the advertised amounts of helpful compounds. Put on your super sleuth hat to find the best products. Use sites like *ConsumerLab.com* or *labdoor.com* for objective evaluations of supplement purity.

Glutathione

Get the edge on Alzheimer's with this awesome antioxidant

It's hard to walk through a grocery store without seeing snacks and drinks that claim to be loaded with antioxidants. But did you know you can actually ramp up your body's natural production of these age-defying compounds?

One such antioxidant — glutathione — can be found in every cell in your body. You need it to fight off free radicals, unstable molecules that can damage your cells. Free radicals are either naturally produced in your body or come from toxins like cigarette smoke and air pollution. If left unchecked, they may increase your risk of dementia and age-related cognitive impairment.

Scientists have found that people with Alzheimer's disease (AD) have lower-than-normal levels of glutathione in the hippocampus — the part of the brain responsible for learning and memory. It's why they think this compound could help fight the progression of dementia. Unfortunately, though, your levels of this antioxidant drop off as you get older.

So what about taking glutathione supplements? Regrettably, they don't easily penetrate the barrier that protects your brain from disease-causing microorganisms in your blood. So researchers looked for an alternative. And they may have found it in N-acetylcysteine, an antioxidant that helps your cells make glutathione.

In a study, scientists divided 43 people with AD into two groups. One took N-acetylcysteine supplements daily and the other received a placebo. After six months, those who took the supplement showed improvements in their memories. In addition, they scored better on tests that measured their verbal skills.

Of course, talk to your doctor before taking N-acetylcysteine. You can find these supplements at supermarkets or online.

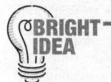

Diet 101: Don't miss out on this superhero of the cell

Your glutathione levels drop as you get older, but supplements aren't the only way to gain them back. All it takes are a few simple tweaks to your diet. So stock up on these foods and vitamins to get more of this important antioxidant.

- Dairy. Researchers who scanned the brains of 60 healthy seniors found that those who got the recommended amount of milk and other dairy products had more glutathione in their brains than those who didn't. Experts say you should aim for at least three servings of dairy a day.

- Sulfur-rich foods. Sulfur is one of the building blocks of glutathione, so foods loaded with this nutrient can help you get more of this antioxidant. Look for cruciferous veggies like broccoli, kale, and cauliflower. Garlic, onions, and other alliums are good sources, too.

- Selenium. Foods like brown rice, Brazil nuts, and cottage cheese are loaded with this powerful mineral. And experts know that getting more selenium in your diet will help ensure you get enough glutathione.

- Vitamin C. Researchers think vitamin C neutralizes free radicals, which helps maintain your supply of glutathione. One study found that healthy adults who took 500 milligrams of vitamin C daily over two weeks increased the amount of glutathione in their red blood cells by 47%.

Step up to better health with glutathione

Want to keep a car running for decades? You'll need to pay attention to more than just the radiator. If you don't keep up with oil changes, for example, your engine may get damaged. And your body isn't all that different. If you're not careful, complications from diabetes and liver disease can extend to your brain. Fortunately, glutathione can help you keep your mind and body in great shape.

> Long-term use of glutathione supplements may cause your zinc levels to drop, which could lead to poor appetite, a weak immune system, and other health problems. Talk to your physician if you're considering taking glutathione.

This antioxidant keeps diabetes damage at bay. Studies suggest that people with uncontrolled type 2 diabetes have less glutathione in their bodies. Experts think that's because they have low levels of two amino acids — cysteine and glycine — that are needed to produce this powerful antioxidant.

So it's not surprising to learn that a study of adults with uncontrolled type 2 diabetes found that those who took daily cysteine and glycine supplements raised their glutathione levels after just two weeks. They also saw significant decreases in diabetes-related oxidative stress — an imbalance of free radicals and antioxidants that can harm cells.

Need another reason to keep diabetes under control? The condition can damage your blood vessels and hamper oxygen flow to your brain.

Stop liver disease with glutathione supplements. Nonalcoholic fatty liver disease (NAFLD) refers to a number of conditions in which too much fat is stored in your liver cells. Obesity and type 2 diabetes increase your risk of this disease. Fortunately, glutathione supplements may help treat NAFLD — a condition linked to attention problems, fuzzy memory, and a loss of brain volume.

In a small study, adults with NAFLD spent three months improving their diet and exercise habits. Then they took 300 milligrams of glutathione every day for four months. When tested at the end of the trial, the participants had lower levels of alanine aminotransferase (ALT) — an enzyme that gets released into the blood of people who have liver damage. The scientists say the drop in ALT suggests that glutathione supplements are a potential treatment of NAFLD.

Gotu kola

This tiger soothes you from head to toe

A soothing tiger? Definitely not the four-legged kind you see at the zoo. This tiger is actually tiger grass, a nickname for the herb gotu kola — pronounced just the way it looks. Legend has it that tigers in the wild rub their wounds on this Asian plant to help them heal. So following their lead, popular skin care brands are adding gotu kola to their moisturizers and anti-aging serums. But there's more to this herb than just a pretty face.

Gotu kola is a commonly eaten leafy green that's popular in southeast Asian countries. You'll find it in juices, drinks, and other food products native to the region because it contains lots of nutrients everyone needs — including vitamin C, various B vitamins, proteins, and minerals.

Popularly known as the "herb of longevity" — got to love that name — gotu kola is a low-growing perennial that lives in warm, tropical climates. This plant has played an important role in traditional medicine for centuries.

Practitioners claim gotu kola can heal skin issues. Not just tigers'. Yours, too. And they say it can boost your brainpower. Here's what the research says.

Ever heard the saying "too much sugar for a dime?" It means something is more trouble than it's worth. That can be the case with some people and gotu kola. The herb may cause problems like sleepiness or liver damage. Steer clear of gotu kola if you're taking sedatives or have liver disease. Questions? Ask your doctor.

This ancient herb perks up your mood. In a small study, two 500-milligram (mg) capsules of gotu kola were given daily over two months to adults with generalized anxiety disorder (GAD). People who have GAD worry excessively about common events and situations. No other medications used to treat anxiety, including antidepressants, were allowed.

- At the end of the study, the participants had lower levels of stress, anxiety, and depression.

- They also reported an improved quality of life.

- And there were no side effects like vertigo, nausea, or dizziness — common complaints with other medications.

Upgrade your memory with this green plant. A study of seniors with mild cognitive impairment found that scores measuring their cognitive function improved after taking 500 mg of gotu kola twice a day for six months.

But that's not all. The researchers also found improvements in other age-related conditions like high blood pressure, constipation, insomnia, and loss of appetite.

A separate study of people who had suffered strokes found that gotu kola extract was just as effective as folic acid in improving cognitive function in people suffering from vascular cognitive impairment. Folic acid has commonly been used to treat the condition.

What's more, the scientists say, gotu kola worked better than folic acid in improving memory. They attributed the results of the study, in part, to gotu kola's antioxidant and anti-inflammatory properties.

> Gotu kola, your new go-to tea. Add 1 teaspoon of finely chopped dried or fresh gotu kola leaves to 1 cup of hot water. Cover the cup and steep for 10 to 15 minutes. If you prefer a stronger flavor, steep the leaves longer. Add your favorite herbs or honey to taste. Strain the tea, if desired.

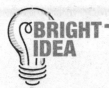

BRIGHT IDEA

DIY herbal healing:
How to grow gotu kola

Ready to give gotu kola a try? Grow your own with these tried-and-true tips.

You can buy gotu kola seeds or plants at local garden centers or online. Here's how to get started if you want to grow your plant from a seedling.

Fill a container with lightweight potting soil. Make sure your pot has a hole in the bottom for drainage. After you plant the seeds, water thoroughly. Move the seedlings into individual containers when they have produced at least one set of true leaves. Those are the second set of leaves that form after the seedling has sprouted.

Allow the young plants to mature for several months, watering just enough to keep the soil moist. Gotu kola grows well in a shallow pot with a plate underneath to keep the soil damp.

Another option? Transplant your gotu kola to your garden when you're sure there won't be any more frost. If your soil contains lots of clay or is compact, add compost, coarse sand, or partially composted pine bark. Gotu kola grows best when the soil is kept moist and has good drainage.

In mild climates, grow gotu kola in full sun. But in hotter places, plant gotu kola in a spot that gets sun in the morning and shade in the afternoon.

When your gotu kola is ready for harvest, put those leaves to good use. Enjoy this herb as an addition to your tossed salad. Or blend it with fruits and veggies — including apple, kale, ginger, and lemon — when juicing.

Grapes

This fantastic fruit can juice up your mind

Could the secret to keeping your brain youthful, preserving your memory, and staving off Alzheimer's and dementia be hiding in your grocery store? The humble grape could hold the key to keeping your mind in tiptop shape.

Go grape to defend against Alzheimer's disease. Grape juice is loaded with resveratrol — a naturally occurring compound that experts say may impact cognitive decline.

In a small study, people with mild or moderate Alzheimer's disease (AD) were asked to take a resveratrol supplement or a placebo every day. After a year, researchers examined the brains of all the participants. They discovered that the resveratrol group showed little or no change in Alzheimer's markers in their brains, but those who took the placebo showed signs that the disease was still progressing.

Some people in the study were taking up to 2,000 milligrams of resveratrol a day, which is impossible to get through your diet. You'd have to drink over 2,000 glasses of grape juice to come close. Fortunately, early research suggests that eating a realistic amount of grapes may help protect you from AD, too.

The small study, published in *Experimental Gerontology*, found that eating grape powder — equivalent to 2 1/4 cups of grapes a day — for six months slowed decline in areas of the brain related to Alzheimer's in people with early memory problems.

Charge up your memory with this powerful drink. A study, published in *The American Journal of Clinical Nutrition*, found grape juice can help improve cognitive function and memory.

In the small trial, women were asked to drink a 12-ounce glass of Concord grape juice or a nearly identical-tasting sugar-sweetened drink every day for three months. Researchers tested aspects of cognitive function, including verbal and spatial memory, attention, and driving performance.

Then, after a four-week washout period, the women switched drinks and repeated the experiment. Researchers found the women had better spatial memory and driving performance after drinking juice. Experts think that's because grape flavonoids may increase activity in the hippocampus, the part of your brain involved in processing spatial memories.

Double down on this drink to reap juicy rewards

The first juice box was introduced in 1974 by a Swedish inventor named Ruben Rausing. Before long, little boxes of fruit juice were a staple in every lunchbox in America. But if you think of juice as just a schoolyard staple, you might want to think again. Research says this powerful drink could help you manage your cholesterol, fight off gum disease, and even de-stress.

Go for white grape juice to give your good cholesterol a helping hand. Scientists recently discovered that an ice-cold glass of grape juice could help you raise your good cholesterol level.

In the study, researchers asked women between the ages of 50 and 67 to drink white grape juice every day for a month. And at the end of the study, they were slimmer and had higher levels of HDL cholesterol.

This good cholesterol carries extra cholesterol to your liver, where it's broken down and filtered out of your body. And that's great for your brain. If your cholesterol is too high, it can block the arteries leading to your brain. That increases your risk of having a stroke and developing dementia or Alzheimer's disease.

Want to try it yourself? People in the study were told to drink 7 milliliters of juice a day for every kilogram they weighed. For someone weighing 160 pounds, that works out to a bit more than 2 cups a day.

Call on red grapes to save your smile. White grape juice isn't the only type you should keep in your pantry. Red grape juice is loaded with resveratrol. Experts say this polyphenol can help fight inflammation in your arteries, which lowers your risk of heart disease. So it's probably no surprise that resveratrol may also battle the inflammation that can lead to chronic gum infections known as periodontitis.

> Winemaking leaves behind piles of grape skins, seeds, and pulp. Traditionally, wineries compost the leftovers or just throw everything away. However, these byproducts are still rich in polyphenols and antioxidants, so people have found ways to turn their trash into healthy nutritional supplements and grapeseed oil.

In fact, Brazilian researchers recently published a review of 11 studies that show resveratrol may slow the progression of gum disease. And putting the brakes on that condition is important to keeping your brain healthy. Research suggests the same bacteria that cause gum infections may contribute to the buildups of plaques found in the brains of people with Alzheimer's disease.

Sit back and sip on this relaxing drink. Had a long day? You might want to pour yourself a soothing glass of juice. Early research suggests resveratrol may affect a compound called phosphodiesterase 4 (PDE4), which is connected to the control of stress in the brain.

Animal studies link high amounts of PDE4 to symptoms of depression and anxiety, but resveratrol helped block the expression of the compound. Cheers!

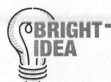

BRIGHT IDEA

Jazz up your grapes with these kitchen hacks

Tired of eating grapes on their own or tossing them into a fruit salad? Try these surprisingly simple tricks to find a new spin on this old fruit.

- Roast your grapes for a sweet treat. Preheat your oven to 425 degrees and toss your grapes with olive oil, salt, and pepper. Roast them on a foil-lined baking sheet for about 30 minutes. The grapes will get jammy and extra sweet, which makes them perfect in a salad, as a side dish, or even as a topping for ice cream.

- Use your freezer to make this healthy summer snack. Craving a popsicle? You can freeze a few grapes for a healthier way to indulge on hot days. Simply take clean, dry grapes and put them in an airtight bag or container in your freezer. Let them freeze for a few hours and enjoy.

- Whip up this super salad dressing with your blender. You might sprinkle a few grapes into your salad, but why not try transforming them into a dressing instead? Take a handful of grapes and blend them with olive oil, pepper, and rosemary. If you're not a rosemary fan, try adding other herbs and spices to find your favorite flavor combination.

- Swap out tomatoes to spice up your salsa. Next time you're craving salsa, try combining chopped grapes with some diced onion, cilantro, and lime juice. It's great served with chips or toasted bread.

Green tea

Steep yourself in the brain-building, mood-boosting benefits of tea

An English gentleman in the 19th century had to be on his best behavior when taking tea with a lady. One indelicate move as he put down his spoon and he might not be invited back. You don't have to keep up with old-fashioned etiquette, but if you want a sharper brain as you get older, you may want to make teatime a new tradition.

Drinking green tea is like sipping from the mythical "fountain of youth." It actually protects your brain cells from aging. In fact, in one study, folks over 70 who drank 2 or more cups daily lowered their risk of brain impairment by 54%, compared to those who drank a cup up to three times weekly. Why not try it for yourself?

Long-standing tea traditions favor a healthy brain. People who enjoy a cuppa — as the English say — of green tea on a regular basis could see big benefits.

Researchers asked 957 Chinese seniors about their tea-drinking habits and then monitored their brain function for several years. They found that regular tea drinkers — especially those with a genetic risk for Alzheimer's disease — were less likely to develop brain disorders than those who usually didn't drink tea.

What's the brain connection? Green, black, and oolong tea contain compounds like catechins and L-theanine that may protect your brain from blood vessel and neuron damage through anti-inflammatory and antioxidant activity.

You can't buy happiness, but you can buy tea — and that's good for your mood. Sure, sipping a cozy mug — or a cool glass — of tea makes you feel a little happier. But does science back that up? In fact, it does. In a meta-analysis of 11 studies, scientists found a lower risk for depression among green tea drinkers.

Antidepressant medications target specific chemical imbalances, but health-promoting elements in tea like EGCG (epigallocatechin gallate), other catechins, and L-theanine help your body in several ways. They support multiple networks in your brain that influence depression, including the stress response, inflammatory response, and communication between the gut and brain.

> You'll find no shortage of advice on making your brain work better. But give your organ some credit. The work it does for you is staggering — and it only uses about 400 calories a day.

L-theanine, in particular, is a rising star in recent research. This amino acid gives tea its savory umami flavor. A review of nine studies linked L-theanine to reduced stress and anxiety. The researchers suggest that 200 to 400 milligrams a day of L-theanine as a supplement could help people cope better under stressful conditions.

Take some tea to bolster brain connections. You might be able to strengthen communication between the nerves in your brain with green tea. That's what researchers discovered when they gave 12 healthy men a soft drink containing green tea extract or a placebo. The men completed memory tasks while inside a brain scanner. Those given green tea extract performed significantly better on the memory tasks and showed increased connectivity in certain brain areas.

Another study says drinking tea at least four times a week for about 25 years improved the efficiency of brain connections in seniors. What does that mean? Lead researcher, Assistant Professor Feng Lei from the National University of Singapore, puts it this way.

"Take the analogy of road traffic as an example — consider brain regions as destinations, while the connections between brain regions are roads," he says. "When a road system is better organized, the movement of vehicles and passengers is more efficient and uses less resources. Similarly, when the connections between brain regions are more structured, information processing can be performed more efficiently."

Play it cool — get more antioxidant power with a cold brew

The grass may look greener on the other side of the street. No matter. Your cold-brew green tea can be greener than your neighbor's hot-brew green tea because your method preserves your tea's chlorophyll.

Need another reason to cold brew your tea? Steeping in cold water rewards you with less bitterness than you get preparing it hot. What's even better is that brewing in your refrigerator holds on to more of those healthy antioxidants like EGCG.

The secret to the best cold-brew quart of green tea is found in the leaves. Choose high-quality, loose-leaf organic tea. Lab tests have shown that you get more EGCG from loose leaves. Tea connoisseurs recommend a spring or "first-harvest" variety. Make sure you store it in an airtight canister or bag and use it within six months for the best flavor.

- Start with a glass or plastic container, and add a quart of filtered or bottled water.

- Drop a heaping tablespoon of tea leaves into your water. You can make the tea stronger or weaker by adjusting the amount of leaves.

- Place your container in the refrigerator for about eight hours. Do this before bedtime and you can sip on your tea throughout the next day. Be sure to strain the leaves out first.

Green tea goes the distance to keep you healthy

Eleanor Roosevelt was rumored to have said, "A woman is like a tea bag — you can't tell how strong she is until you put her in hot water." Women and men alike need courage to face serious health conditions, but they have a friend in the fight.

Green tea brings heavyweight antioxidant power to the ring. It helps knock down ailments and reinforce your immune system. In fact, it may be possible to prevent three of the top killer ailments — heart disease, cancer, and stroke — and more with this powerful drink.

Healthier hearts prefer green tea. At least that's what green tea-drinking habits of more than 90,000 Japanese people age 40 to 69 suggests. Compared to people who drank less than 1 cup of tea daily, regular tea drinkers had a lower risk of dying early from heart disease.

Researchers think the reason could be because catechins in green tea like epigallocatechin gallate (EGCG) act as antioxidants to help lower blood pressure and control body fat. That's good news since research has linked high blood pressure to memory loss and a reduced ability to think quickly.

> Communities of microbes come together in your mouth to create a biofilm so they can hide from your immune system and antimicrobial agents like toothpaste. Their activity sets you up for a nasty oral infection. But green tea polyphenols may stop the biofilm from forming on your teeth in the first place.

Sip your green tea and tell cancer to take a hike. Green tea may be the ultimate fighting champion when it comes to the big C. In fact, it could lower your risk of developing breast cancer, according to a review of 14 studies involving 29,101 women.

A green tea bob and weave dodges stroke. In a classic matchup, more than 83,000 Japanese adults age 45 to 74 told researchers how often they drank green tea, if at all. After 13 years, the record was clear. The more green tea people drank, the lower their risk was of dying from stroke.

Bad cholesterol is no match for green tea. Low-density lipoprotein (LDL) is the cholesterol you don't want hanging around because it puts you at higher risk for rapid cognitive decline. But green tea catechins may send LDL packing, says a meta-analysis.

Daily green tea supplements ranging from 145 to 3,000 milligrams a day given to participants for three to 24 weeks lowered total and LDL cholesterol compared to controls. Experts believe this effect was likely due to the antioxidants in green tea.

Looking for an accountability partner in weight loss, ladies? Green tea extract could help you slim down. In a study, 102 over-weight or obese women took a high-dose green tea extract or a placebo daily for 12 weeks.

- The green tea group experienced weight loss and a lower BMI.

- Their waistlines shrunk compared to the placebo group, too.

And that's great for their overall health because conditions arising from obesity, including diabetes, high blood pressure, and heart disease, can negatively affect your brain.

Hearing aids

Hear how to protect against dementia and depression

Do you often ask people to repeat themselves? Has it become a struggle to talk over the phone? Maybe loved ones complain that your television is too loud. If so, you already have a lot in common with about 1 in 3 adults between the ages of 65 and 74 — that's how widespread hearing problems are. Nearly half of folks older than 75 are in the same boat.

But you don't have to be one of them. Help your sound sensors, and you may ward off depression and dementia.

Amplify brain health when you help your ears. You may not be surprised that hearing loss can damage your relationships. After all, socializing can be frustrating and embarrassing if you can't participate in a conversation. But disconnecting from these interactions means you miss out on stimulation that's key to healthy brain function. The stress of distancing yourself can even increase inflammation in your body and make your brain more vulnerable to the damaging effects of Alzheimer's disease.

However, you may delay the onset of dementia and more with hearing aids. During a recent study, researchers followed a group of nearly 115,000 people age 66 and older with newly diagnosed hearing loss.

- In the three years following diagnosis, the seniors who wore hearing aids had a lower risk of Alzheimer's disease compared to people whose hearing loss was left uncorrected.

- The risk of being diagnosed with anxiety and depression or having a fall-related injury was also lower for participants with devices.

Save your social life and your brain — who wouldn't go for that? But only a small percentage of people with a hearing loss diagnosis actually get hearing aids. If you decide to be one of the few, you may have a better health outcome.

Protect your mind at the speed of sound by getting tested. Hearing loss can come from external sources, like long-term exposure to loud sounds, or internal ones, like high blood pressure or diabetes. And your hearing can gradually worsen as you age, so you may not notice any changes at first.

Unlike many risk factors for dementia and depression, though, hearing loss is treatable. That's why it's important for you to get tested regularly.

Audiologists and ear-nose-throat (ENT) doctors can usually diagnose the cause of your hearing loss. Looking for a quick hearing check that doesn't require an appointment? Lots of hearing aid manufacturers — Miracle-Ear, Phonak, Oticon, and Signia, to name a few — offer free online assessments. Just remember you should have a professional check your hearing each year if you're age 60 or older.

Want to connect with other people who live with hearing loss? Get plugged into a support group at *hearingloss.org*, powered by the Hearing Loss Association of America. Poke around the site to find tools on living with hearing loss and news about the latest technological and medical advances.

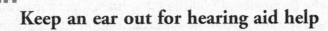

BRIGHT IDEA

Keep an ear out for hearing aid help

Left untreated, hearing loss can lead to depression and social isolation. So why do only 20% of people who could benefit from hearing aids use them? Sticker shock is a major reason. A single hearing aid, on average, fetches $2,400. That's close to $5,000 a pair. And original Medicare won't cover the cost. Luckily, there are organizations ready to help so you can get aids without busting your bank account.

- If you've served in the U.S. military, call your nearest Veterans Administration (VA) and ask for the Veterans Service Center to find out if you qualify for free hearing aids.

- Some states cover hearing services for adults under their Medicaid programs. Find your state's Medicaid office contact info at *medicaid.gov/about-us/contact-us/contact-state-page.html*.

- Many local Lions Clubs offer affordable hearing aids to individuals based on their income. Go to *lionsclubs.org* and click the "Find a Club" button to locate your nearest club and get an application.

- The Starkey Hearing Foundation supplies hearing aids to people who otherwise can't afford them. Visit *starkeyhearingfoundation.org/hearing-assistance* or call 800-328-8602 to speak with a consultant about the Hear Now program.

- The nonprofit AUDIENT assists low-income seniors in finding hearing aids and related treatments at deep discounts. Call 866-956-5400, ext. 2 to speak with a representative.

- Visit Hearing Charities of America at *hearingaiddona-tions.org/resources* for local and national resources.

3 ways to turn down hearing loss

Although the escapades of Charlie Chaplin, Lillian Gish, and other film stars of the early 1900s are entertaining on the big screen, you don't want your life to turn into a silent movie. Keep the sound in your world turned on, and you won't even need hearing aids. These three tips can help you on your way.

Load up on veggies to keep trouble out of earshot. It turns out that when free radicals — rogue molecules that damage healthy cells — form in your inner ear, they magnify your chances of hearing loss.

But you can avoid falling victim. Scientists have learned that people who eat healthy amounts of magnesium and antioxidants, like beta carotene and vitamin C, can hear tones and frequencies better.

So head over to the produce aisle. It's where you'll find beta carotene-packed foods, like sweet potatoes and cantaloupe, and citrus fruits loaded with vitamin C. Mix up your meals with magnesium-heavy green leafy vegetables like kale, collard greens, and spinach.

And don't forget about iron. Researchers have found an association between hearing loss and iron deficiency anemia (IDA) in American adults. But IDA is easy to treat. Fill up with iron-packed leafy greens like spinach and Swiss chard, potatoes with their skin still on, and legumes including soybeans and lentils.

Make a splash by matching delish dishes with ear-soothing sides. Don't forget to pair up some fresh fish and healthy oils with those veggies. That's the advice of researchers who followed the eating patterns of more than 70,000 women in the Nurses' Health Study II over two decades.

The result? Those who followed either a Mediterranean diet — heavy in extra-virgin olive oil, whole grains, fish, and vegetables — or the veggie-rich, low-sodium DASH diet saw the best results. In fact, they had about a 30% lower risk of hearing loss compared to those who adopted less healthy dining habits.

"Eating well contributes to overall good health, and it may also be helpful in reducing the risk of hearing loss," says study co-author Dr. Sharon Curhan, an epidemiologist at Brigham and Women's Hospital.

Slip on your sneakers to score benefits between the ears.
Who would have thought that walking a little over 15 minutes a
day could improve your hearing? But it's true. Scientists in Boston
found that women who walked two or more hours a week lowered
their chances of hearing loss by 10% to 15%, compared to those
who walked less than one hour each week.

Why is walking good for your ears? Physical activity boosts blood
flow throughout your body, which helps keep your arteries relaxed
and flexible. And by controlling your weight with exercise, your
blood vessels are less likely to be damaged by inflammation. That's
good news because better blood flow to your inner ears and less
damage equals a lower risk of hearing loss.

"Hearing loss can impair activities of everyday life, causing frustration,
loneliness, social isolation, and dependence," says Dr. Curhan, co-
author of the study. "We often think of hearing loss as an inevitable
part of the aging process, but these findings provide evidence that
potentially modifiable risk factors, such as maintaining a healthy
weight and staying physically active, may help in the prevention of
hearing loss or delay its progression."

Beware this shocking cause of hearing loss

Loud noise is one of the most common sources of hearing loss.
But you may be surprised to learn that medication can hurt your
ears, too. Aspirin is one of these hidden culprits.

If taken in too high a dose or too often, aspirin can cause ringing
in the ear, called tinnitus, and hearing loss. This is usually tempo-
rary. But sometimes taking aspirin at a high dose for a long period
can lead to permanent damage to your ears.

You should also keep an ear out for other ototoxic medications —
drugs that may harm your ears. For instance, antibiotics like gen-
tamicin or the painkiller Vicodin. Usually, tinnitus is the first sign
your hearing is being impacted. You may also experience hearing
loss or balance problems. These issues may go away when you stop
taking the medication. Other times, the inner ear damage remains.

Your best bet? Ask your doctor if alternative drugs will do the trick. If the ototoxic meds are unavoidable, get baseline hearing and balance tests before you start treatment and stay vigilant about any changes you experience.

Ring up hearing perks by snubbing your cellphone

Can your cellphone habit hurt your hearing? Maybe. In a recent study from India, scientists compared the hearing levels of volunteers who spent different lengths of time on their cellphones.

They discovered that 10% of the group using their mobiles more than an hour a day experienced hearing loss. That compares with 2% in the group who used their phones less than an hour a day. And those who rarely used a cellphone? None reported hearing loss.

The researchers believe long-term and frequent exposure to your cellphone's electromagnetic field damages cells in your inner ear, leading to high-frequency hearing loss. Once that occurs, it's difficult to hear high-pitched sounds like the beeping of your microwave.

What can you do? Experts recommend texting and using a speakerphone, landline, or Bluetooth headset. Keep calls short if you have to hold a phone up to your ear.

Kiwi

Put pep in your step by snacking on this exotic fruit

Want to tone down anger and anxiety, get a bump in energy, and drop your risk of depression? Grab a kiwi. It's packed with two nutrients that will help you improve your mood and crank up your get-up-and-go.

Serve up kiwi to get more vitamin C. Dr. James Lind was one of the first scientists to champion vitamin C, even though he didn't realize it. He discovered citrus could cure sailors of scurvy. However, it took hundreds of years before scientists realized that vitamin C was responsible for those healing powers. And now, experts say this vitamin can do more than support sailors.

A small study published in the *Journal of Nutritional Science* claims that kiwis are some of the best mood boosters you can find. Researchers gave men a questionnaire to rate their anger, anxiety, depression, and energy. Then they asked some of the participants to eat half a kiwi a day, while the others were told to have two kiwis a day.

After six weeks, they rated their moods again. And they found that those who ate two kiwis lowered their depressive symptoms by 32%. Plus they had better overall mood scores. However, those who ate only half a kiwi didn't get enough nutrients see any improvement.

The authors claim the results are due to the vitamin C found in kiwis, which helps improve the levels of dopamine, a chemical messenger in your brain involved in motivation, reward, and attention.

Can't find kiwis at your local grocery store? Experts say people in this study got about 212 milligrams (mg) of vitamin C every day from the two fruits. That's a little more than what you'd find in two large oranges.

Fruit fiber may help keep depression at bay. A single kiwi, without the skin, has 2.7 grams of fiber. And that's good news if you want to fight off depression. Recent research shows that a diet high in fruits and vegetables is one of the best ways to beat back the blues.

> Want to get more fiber? Don't peel your kiwi. The skin is perfectly edible, and it's loaded with extra nutrients. Experts say that simply eating the kiwi's peel can boost the fiber content of the fruit by nearly 50%. Not a fan of the fuzzy texture? Rub it off with a cloth after washing.

A study of 16,807 adults found that people who ate the most fiber from fruits and veggies were about 40% less likely to suffer from depression. Those who ate the highest amount of cereal fibers — from foods like pasta or bread — didn't get the same benefits.

Experts say men over 50 need around 30 grams of fiber every day, and women over 50 need 21 grams.

Triple threat — 1 sweet way to fight 3 major complaints

When the Chinese gooseberry first hit shelves in America, shoppers were wary of the small, fuzzy fruit. The New Zealand agricultural industry decided to rename the fruit after their country's national bird — the kiwi. Now, shoppers love kiwis for their sweet flavor and health benefits. Research suggest this exotic treat can help you fend off these three diseases.

Choose the right fruits to beat high blood pressure. You probably know that a healthy diet can help you lower your blood pressure. But if you pick the right foods, you can get even more protection. Researchers think the kiwi may be a great choice for people with high blood pressure.

Norwegian researchers asked people with high blood pressure to either eat three kiwis or one apple every day. Eight weeks later, they found that those who ate the kiwis had lowered their blood pressure more than the apple eaters. Experts think kiwi's antioxidants help fight off damage that can lead to high blood pressure.

Keeping your blood pressure down isn't just good for your heart. Research shows that high blood pressure can damage the brain's white matter, the tissue that transmits signals between nerve cells.

Keep your cholesterol under control with a few servings of kiwi. Want to protect your brain? You need to keep your arteries clear. When your blood vessels become clogged with cholesterol, your brain doesn't get enough oxygen. Brain cells begin to die and you experience problems like short-term memory loss.

A recent study suggests that keeping your cholesterol in check could be as simple as eating kiwi every week. The researchers examined the diet habits of 1,469 healthy adults and measured their blood lipids and cholesterol levels.

They discovered that people who reported eating at least one kiwi each week were more likely to have higher levels of good cholesterol — the kind that ferries other forms of cholesterol from your blood-stream — and lower blood levels of a type of fat called triglycerides.

Tummy troubles? Opt for a soothing snack. Irritable bowel syndrome can cause constipation, bloating, and stomach pain. And it can even impair your memory and ability to focus on things.

A new study revealed that kiwi extract can help fight off constipation, abdominal pain, and other IBS symptoms. Researchers asked people to either take 2,160 milligrams (mg) of green kiwi extract or a placebo every day for a week.

At the end of the study, the extract group showed improvement in their symptoms compared to the placebo. Experts think the extract helps the helpful bacteria in your gut grow and flourish, which improves digestion.

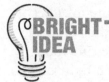

Ripen kiwi quickly with these kitchen hacks

Kiwis don't change color when they ripen, so it can be tricky to tell if they're ready to eat. You have to test them with a gentle squeeze. If the fruits are a bit soft and yield to slight pressure, they're ready to go. But if you have a kiwi that's too firm, don't worry. You can speed up the ripening process with these simple tips.

- Store it with another fruit. Apples and bananas both give off ethylene gas, which is a hormone that causes plants to ripen. Store an apple or banana with an unripe kiwi in a paper bag to help trap the gas and speed up the ripening process.

- Cover it with rice. Don't have a spare paper bag on hand? You can store a kiwi in a tub of uncooked rice instead. Rice will help trap ethylene gas naturally produced by the fruit and speed up the ripening process. Plus you can still use the rice after your kiwi is ready to eat.

- Keep it toasty. Heat helps speed up chemical reactions, like ripening. Keep your kiwi somewhere warm, like on the windowsill or near a vent blowing warm air.

- Use your microwave. Want to ripen fruit even faster? Microwave it on medium heat for about 15 seconds. After that, stick it in a paper bag with the apple or banana, and check it daily to see if it's ready to eat.

L-carnitine

High steaks: Refresh memory and mood with this meaty nutrient

Travel back in time to ninth grade biology, and see if this question rings a bell. Mitochondria, organelles, and cytoplasm are parts of what basic building block of living things? If you guessed "cell," go to the head of the class. If not, time for a review. And here you thought you finished up all that biology stuff decades ago. Nope. Not if you're interested in steering clear of dementia and depression.

Charge up your cells to fight dementia. Lysosomes are part of a special group of cell structures called organelles. It's their job to store the enzymes that change amino acids into L-carnitine. Then L-carnitine helps move fatty acids in the cytoplasm — the jello-like fluid in your cells — into the mitochondria, the cell power plant that burns the fats as energy. It's true your body can make its own L-carnitine, but for medical or genetic reasons, some people can't. So for them, getting enough can be an issue.

Researchers know there are several forms of carnitine, but acetyl-L-carnitine (ALC) may be the most effective kind for firing up your brain. They say ALC is absorbed more efficiently than other forms of carnitine so more gets into your brain tissue.

In one study, 56 seniors with vascular dementia were given cognitive tests. Then they were divided into two groups. One group took 500 milligrams (mg) of ALC three times a day for 28 weeks. The other was given a placebo. At the end of the study, researchers found that the folks given ALC performed better on attention and language tests than the control group.

The scientists who ran the study didn't provide a reason for the results. But separate research suggests ALC improves how well the mito-chondria in your brain function, something that declines with age.

Depressed? Try a little ALC. Researchers looked back on a dozen studies involving nearly 800 adults and found that those who were given ALC supplements experienced fewer symptoms of depression than those who took placebos. And in studies comparing ALC to antidepressants, ALC showed similar effectiveness in reducing symptoms. The researchers found that ALC appeared to work best in older adults.

Boost ALC through your diet.
How much ALC do you need? There are no dietary reference intakes or recommended daily allowances for L-carnitine. But most adults who eat mixed diets with red meat and other animal products take in about 60 to 180 mg per day.

Researchers warn that supplements of 3,000 mg or more each day may cause side effects like nausea and vomiting.

What foods contain the most L-carnitine? Remember this. The redder the meat, the higher the amount. Four ounces of steak can supply 162 milligrams (mg). The same amount of ground beef? Up to 99 mg. You'll also get 8 mg in 1 cup of whole milk. Or 3 mg in 1/2 cup of delicious ice cream.

Put an end to broken hearts and stop the sugar blues

Remember singing along to the Bee Gees as they crooned their 1970s hit, "How Can You Mend a Broken Heart?" Maybe your musical memories go even further back, all the way to the 1950s with the McGuire Sisters warbling their way through "Sugartime."

Remember the lyrics? "Sugar in the mornin', sugar in the evenin', sugar at suppertime."

But what do these two golden oldies have in common? A verse of each ditty should have featured lyrics about L-carnitine. It's one powerful nutrient — and antioxidant — that could take out both heart disease and high blood sugar.

L-carnitine can get your heart on the mend. Ever hear of oxidative stress? It's an imbalance between free radicals — unstable and highly reactive molecules that can damage your cells — and the antioxidants that fight them. It's important, because those rogue and highly excitable molecules can cause heart disease.

So what's a body to do? L-carnitine to the rescue. In a small study of seniors with cardiovascular disease, half of the participants received 1,000 milligrams of L-carnitine daily for 12 weeks. The other half took a placebo. At the end of the study, blood tests showed an increase in antioxidative enzymes in the people who took the L-carnitine.

That's a positive sign, the researchers say, because low levels of antioxidative enzymes have been linked to a narrowing of the arteries that lead to your heart.

This nutrient helps you pass all your exams. If you know anything about diabetes, you're probably familiar with these tests.

- Fasting plasma glucose (FPG) measures a person's sugar level after they haven't eaten for at least eight hours.

- HbA1C test measures your average blood sugar over the past two to three months.

People with diabetes need to keep their blood sugar levels under control to avoid other health complications, including nerve damage and memory loss. And it appears L-carnitine may help. A review of dozens of studies on glycemic control found that people who took L-carnitine supplements had significantly lower FPG, insulin levels, and HbA1C concentrations than those in control groups.

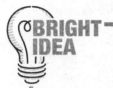

Beef up your L-carnitine levels with the right stuff

You're concerned about developing dementia, or maybe you've experienced a few symptoms of depression. After talking to your doctor, you both agree that an L-carnitine supplement might work for you. Here's a quick guide to help you — and your doctor — decide which supplement would be the right choice.

- Acetyl-L-carnitine, also known as Alcar, is the most effective for your brain. It is sold over the counter without a prescription. Acetyl-L-carnitine helps produce acetylcholine, a chemical compound that plays an important role in memory and cognition. Severe depletion of acetylcholine is associated with Alzheimer's disease. Supplemental doses usually range from 0.5 to 2 grams per day.

- Propionyl-L-carnitine helps high blood pressure and circulatory problems like peripheral vascular disease, a disorder that can cause the blood vessels outside your heart and brain to narrow. Propionyl-L-carnitine may help produce nitric oxide, which improves blood flow. Propionyl-L-carnitine is not approved by the FDA for use as a drug to treat any condition, but it's sold over the counter as a nutritional supplement. Ask your medical professional about the correct usage of this product.

- L-carnitine L-tartrate is used to help sore muscles recover after exercise. It also transports fat into your cells. Once there, the fat can be used for energy. L-cartinine L-tartrate is sold online, at health food stores, and over the counter. Doses may vary from 1 to 4 grams per day, depending on your need and your doctor's advice.

Laughter

Go ahead and bust a gut — it's good medicine for your mind

Think back to your favorite Frankie Avalon and Annette Funicello beach flick from the 1960s. Can't you just see them smiling from ear to ear? Turns out that kind of beaming, joyful grin is called a Duchenne smile. It's different from a polite, social smile because it puts a lot more of your facial muscles to work, especially those around your eyes.

A broad grin makes you feel good. And the laughter that comes with it does more than improve your mood. It benefits your mind.

Laugh off stress? It's no joke. An old expression says, "He who laughs last, laughs longest." Who doesn't want to live longer? Here's how a sense of humor can help.

Stress causes levels of the hormone cortisol to increase in your blood. That leads to a rise in your heart rate and blood pressure. But laughter lowers cortisol levels, making you feel more relaxed.

Researchers wanted to see if a therapeutic laughter program (TLP) could reduce stress, anxiety, and depression in 60 women undergoing radiation treatment for breast cancer. Half of them participated in four TLP sessions. The other half didn't.

Each hourlong session included relaxation exercises and prolonged periods of laughter. At the end of the study, the TLP group reported lower levels of stress, anxiety, and depression than the control group. Even better, they experienced those benefits after just a single session.

Giggle, cackle, and howl your way to a better memory. When was the last time you had a good, long chuckle? Here's another reason to make room for laughter in your daily routine.

Just 20 minutes of watching a funny video can lower cortisol levels. Those were the findings of researchers who measured the cortisol levels of 20 healthy seniors and then randomly divided them into two groups. One group watched a segment of "America's Funniest Home Videos" or a Red Skelton comedy clip. The other sat quietly without watching anything.

The researchers tested the volunteers' cortisol levels once more and found

> Ever thought of taking a laughing class? Students from the Kalinga Institute of Social Sciences gathered a few years ago in northeastern India to do just that — a whopping 15,991 of them formed the largest laughter yoga class on record. You can learn more about the exercise at *laughteryoga.org*.

they were much lower in the group that had been laughing. Not only that, the video-watching group performed significantly better than the control group on a test that measured their ability to remember a list of words for more than 10 minutes.

So how can chuckling help your memory? Laughter combats stress, which is bad for your short-term memory. It also triggers the release of endorphins and dopamine — two feel-good chemicals — so you feel happier. And guess what happiness does for you? It changes your brain waves, which can improve your memory.

Laugh it up to lower blood sugar and heart disease risk

American editor Norman Cousins wrote that laughter helped him survive a life-threatening disease. He called it a kind of "internal exercise" for someone in bed and recovering from an illness. Cousins isn't the only prominent person to have said that gelotology — the study of laughter's effects on the body — is good medicine. But why does laughter work?

Yuck it up and dial back blood sugar. Did you know that clowns dress up as doctors and visit youngsters coping with diseases like diabetes? These clowns give children a welcome pick-me-up that's got real science behind it.

Researchers devised a method to test laughter's effect on blood sugar. They asked healthy seniors and those with type 2 diabetes (T2D) to eat a 500-calorie meal. Both groups then watched a 40-minute humorless lecture. The next day, they ate the same meal and watched a comedy routine. On both days, their blood sugar levels were measured before eating and again two hours later.

Of course, the food sparked an increase in blood sugar in both groups — but much less on the day of the comedy routine. One possible reason? Laughing put the participants' glucose-burning muscles to work. The results were particularly strong in the seniors with T2D. That's good news because high blood sugar can damage blood vessels and restrict blood flow to your brain.

Hearty laughter promotes vascular health. When something strikes your funny bone, you may find yourself gasping for air and slapping your knee. As the guffawing subsides, you feel strangely relaxed. So what happens inside your body when you laugh like that?

A rip-roaring laugh raises your heart and breathing rate, along with your blood pressure. And when you stop, all three cool down. The end result? You feel at ease and laid-back. What's more, laughter causes your pituitary gland to release feel-good hormones called endorphins. These turn on receptors that tell your body to make nitric oxide — a chemical that causes your blood vessels to dilate. This leads to increased blood flow.

In a small study, researchers asked healthy adults to watch 15- to 30-minute segments of stressful and humorous films, a minimum of 48 hours apart. The clips produced very different results. Blood flow in the participants' arms increased during the funny clips and fell during the stressful scenes. In fact, compared with when the volunteers were stressed, some 50% more blood flowed when the participants laughed.

What's the benefit of better blood flow? Less risk of blood clots that can block arteries supplying blood to your heart and brain.

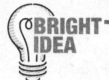

Happy spaces, happy faces make laughter a priority

Oxford University made history in 2015 when it announced its word of the year wasn't a word. It was an emoji. Specifically, the "laughing emoji." You know the one — it's got a wide, toothy grin and eyes that cry tears of joy. People around the globe use it tell others on social media that they find something really funny.

So get your thumb ready. You're going to want to "like" these ways to belly up to some sidesplitting laughter.

- Splurge on funny shows or movies. You can watch these at home, but consider going out with a group to the theater or a comedy show.

- Hang up your favorite comics or funny pictures so you'll see them more often.

- Practice laughing. Take a laughter yoga class for tips, or join a laughing club.

- Mine your experiences for golden nuggets of humor. Share your tales with others.

- Tickle someone. Or, better yet. Let someone tickle you.

- Look up some jokes and try them out on your friends. Even if they're silly, the groans they elicit are worth a chuckle.

- Even annoying moments may be ripe for comedy picking. Whether it's a bed-head hairdo or a coffee splatter on your trousers, turn everyday nuisances into smiles.

Obviously, not everyone finds the same things funny. So remember to be sensitive to people around you when you're experimenting with humor.

Leafy greens

3 powerful nutrients to sharpen your brain

Returning to your "salad days" can be more than a trip down memory lane when you fill up your bowl with leafy greens. These veggies are packed with nutrients that may help ward off dementia and keep your brain young. Your friends will be green with envy when they hear about all the benefits you're gaining.

Push back against dementia with carotenoids. Many of the red, orange, and yellow foods that paint your plate owe their bright color to carotenoids. These pigments are also found in leafy greens, and their purpose isn't just decorative. Eating more of the carotenoids lutein and zeaxanthin is associated with lower cognitive decline.

These two are also the main carotenoids in your brain and are mostly found in areas vulnerable to Alzheimer's disease. So perhaps it's no surprise that, in a study of seniors without dementia, researchers found that participants with higher levels of lutein in their blood had a lower risk of dementia and Alzheimer's.

Folate does double duty for your mind. A sharp brain at 70 — it may be as simple as eating spinach and mustard greens. These foods are high in folate — a nutrient around 75% of Americans don't get enough of. But you can combat dementia, depression, and deficiency by adding more into your diet.

In one study, researchers found that people with the most folate in their diet had an approximately 50% lower risk of dementia than participants who got the least folate.

And that's not the end of folate's powerful influence. In a study following more than 2,000 adults, depression was less common in participants with high folate concentrations compared to those with the lowest levels of folate. That difference is likely due to folate's role in the production of S-adenosylmethionine (SAM). SAM can impact your neurotransmitters and hormones, and an imbalance in these chemicals is associated with depression.

BRIGHT IDEA

Max out the goodness of your greens

Boil leafy green cruciferous vegetables like kale, cabbage, bok choy, and arugula, and you may be pouring health benefits down the drain — literally. That's because you can lose some nutrients in the cooking water or destroy them with heat. But catering your preparation to your greens of choice can help you get more out of them.

For cruciferous veggies, a quick steam or stir-fry will keep their helpful, cancer-fighting glucosinolates intact. Nutrients like folate and vitamin C are also vulnerable during cooking. High heat can impact both, and levels can drop with extended time in water.

However, some greens, like spinach, are actually more nutritious after being cooked. Simply blanching spinach can help your body absorb more calcium and iron.

Pressure cooking may be the best of both worlds. This technique decreases the amount of time your greens spend soaking and exposed to high heat. Try it by putting a layer of water at the bottom of an electric pressure cooker, setting in a metal steaming basket, and dropping your greens in the basket where they'll be out of the water.

Don't get lost in the weeds, though. Your meal as a whole matters because different foods can have surprising interactions. For example, leafy greens are an excellent source of iron, but drinking tea after eating them can cancel out both of their benefits. That's because their nutrients bind to one another, leaving little for you to absorb. A simple trick for this pair is to add lemon to your tea. It makes more iron available for your body.

Vitamin K victuals KO cognitive decline. The fountain of youth may be fantasy, but when it comes to a younger brain, the benefits of leafy greens are research-backed reality. In fact, in a five-year study, people who ate one to two servings of leafy greens every day had the cognitive ability of a person 11 years younger than the people who didn't eat any.

Researchers believe greens such as kale and collards may owe their benefits to nutrients like vitamin K, lutein, folate, and beta carotene.

Other studies back the brain bonuses of vitamin K. One group of researchers found that people age 65 and older who got the most vitamin K in their diets had better scores on tests that measure brain function and dementia-related behavior than those who got the least. That may be because vitamin K influences neuron activity.

> Getting all the nutrients you need from your greens? Think again. If you take NSAIDs like aspirin or ibuprofen, your body may not be absorbing all the available calcium and iron. To avoid deficiencies, take these medications in the smallest dose and shortest amount of time possible.

A trio of troubles? Leaf it to these versatile vegetables

Endive watercress salad, beet green omelet, garlicky sauteed Swiss chard. You'll enjoy tons of ways to load up on leafy greens. Better yet, they're versatile in your body, too — helping your head, heart, and more.

See how leafy greens elevate your eyesight. Did you know that taking good care of your eyes may prevent cognitive decline? Researchers believe poor vision may keep you from taking part in activities that stimulate your mind. But eating your greens may be one way you can protect yourself against major eye conditions like macular degeneration.

This disease develops when the part of your retina called the macula is damaged. The effect is serious — you start to lose your central vision. Luckily, greens may be able to help.

Over 2,000 adults were studied in the 15-year Blue Mountains Eye Study. Researchers found that people who ate 100 to 142 milligrams (mg) of vegetable nitrates every day had a 35% lower risk of developing early signs of macular degeneration compared with people who ate fewer than 69 mg. To put that in context, you might get up to 100 mg of nitrates from about a cup of spinach. Keep in mind, the nitrate content of vegetables is influenced by growth and storage conditions, so amounts can vary greatly.

> Nitrates may also play a role in protecting against glaucoma. In a study of more than 100,000 people, those who ate the most leafy greens had a 20% to 30% lower risk of developing glaucoma than those who ate the least. How much did the veggie lovers polish off? About one and a half servings a day.

"If our findings are confirmed," said lead researcher, Associate Professor Bamini Gopinath, "incorporating a range of foods rich in dietary nitrates — like green leafy vegetables and beetroot — could be a simple strategy to reduce the risk of early macular degeneration."

How does it work? Your body turns dietary nitrates into nitric oxide, which plays an important role in maintaining good blood flow throughout your body, including your eyes.

Hearty greens protect your ticker. Around the world people are jeopardizing their health by not eating enough leafy greens. That's why researchers considered the link between these veggies and heart disease in a review of eight studies. They found that compared to people with the lowest intake, those who ate the most leafy greens had a nearly 16% lower risk of heart disease.

Eating extra greens is the simple solution, but if you want to do even more, try steaming them. Steam cooking improves bile acid-binding activity which ultimately reduces fat absorption — protecting your heart in the process.

But it's more than your heart health at risk. Heart disease can damage your blood vessels and disrupt the flow of oxygen-rich blood to your brain.

Turn over a new leaf in diabetes prevention. Fiber does more than encourage digestive health. It also defends against diabetes by improving your insulin sensitivity and promoting weight loss. Leafy greens are one great source of the fiber you need. Plus they're packed with antioxidants like vitamin C and lutein that may help, too.

All these forces join together to reduce your risk of developing type 2 diabetes. So go green to balance your blood sugar. You'll be supporting your mind, too. That's because diabetes is bad news for your memory. It damages your blood vessels and hampers oxygen flow to your brain.

BRIGHT IDEA

Homegrown goodness: Sow a gourmet salad in your backyard

Spring salad, or mesclun as the French know it, is a refreshing and colorful mix of lettuce, endive, chervil, and arugula leaves. You can easily grow these trendy greens and more.

Just mix together the various seeds and sprinkle them on a prepared bed. Sow only enough seeds to produce greens to feed you for a week. Plant another batch the following week for a continuous harvest.

Once they are a few inches tall, chop down the greens to within an inch of the ground and fertilize the bed. Your greens will be ready to pick again in a month.

Legumes

Pile your plate with beans to protect your brain and heart

Beans, chickpeas, lentils, peas, and soybeans — they're all part of the legume family. And experts are catching on to the fact that legumes are loaded with fiber, protein, and the heart-saving, brain-boosting, stroke-stopping, mood-enhancing vitamin that you absolutely shouldn't miss out on — folate.

Lentils lend a hand in beating the blues. Feeling down? Don't tuck into a bowl of ice cream for a pick-me-up. Instead, dig into a bowl of lentils. A single cup clocks in with 358 micrograms (mcg) of folate. That's 90% of the amount you need each day. Experts think getting enough of this type of B vitamin is key to warding off depression.

Researchers examined the concentration of vitamins in the blood of 2,791 adults. And they found that women with higher levels of folate had less of a risk of depression than those with the lower levels.

Researchers think folate helps your body produce a compound called S-adenosylmethionine, which your body uses to produce mood-boosting chemicals in your brain like dopamine and serotonin.

Want to dodge dementia? Load up on legumes. Folate does more than lift your spirits. Scientists think this nutrient may keep your mind sharp as you age, too.

Researchers looked at the diets of 1,321 seniors. They found that people who ate the most folate every day — 375 mcg or more — had a 50% lower risk of dementia compared to those who ate the least.

The authors of the study think this vitamin helps repair damaged DNA in your brain cells, a process that can help prevent cognitive decline.

Grab a bowl of beans to steer clear of cardiovascular disease and stroke. A recent analysis of 277 trials published in the *Annals of Internal Medicine* found that people who get more folic acid — the man-made version of folate — have a lower risk of stroke.

Pulses — the technical term for the seeds of the legume plant that you eat — are loaded with other nutrients that offer protection, too. A separate review linked increased pulse consumption to a lower risk of cardiovascular disease. The researchers found that 81 grams of pulses a day did the trick. That's a bit less than half a cup.

Experts say the heart-protective effects come from the fiber, magnesium, potassium, and protein in pulses.

> Every cell in your body needs thiamine (vitamin B1). Your nerves use it to carry signals from your brain to other parts of your body. Your heart and muscles also need thiamine to function properly. A cup of black beans boasts 33% of your daily needs.

Lose weight and ditch diabetes with legumes

Legumes have long been seen as poor man's food. During the Great Depression, for example, the government touted beans as a cheap, filling alternative to meat. But now, penny pinchers aren't the only ones eating legumes. Research shows these nutritional powerhouses can help you lose weight and fight diabetes.

Win the battle of the bulge with a protein-packed meal. Want to trim your waistline? Scientists say you should swap out meat for beans and peas. Danish researchers compared the fullness factor of 43 healthy men who ate high-protein breakfast patties made from either peas and beans or veal and pork. The men reported feeling fuller after eating the veggie patties than the meat patties.

What's more, they ate 12% fewer calories at lunch after having eaten the vegetable patties for breakfast. The experts say the high amounts of fiber in the beans and peas probably made the men feel full for longer. Fiber, after all, takes a relatively long time to digest.

Even better, losing weight can help keep your brain healthy in your golden years. That's because obesity raises your risk of developing conditions linked to dementia, including heart disease and type 2 diabetes.

Load up on this mighty mineral to control blood sugar.
Diabetes is bad news for your memory. It damages your blood vessels and hampers oxygen flow to your brain. In addition, spikes in blood sugar also damage brain cells. So if you're at risk for diabetes, it's a good idea to make sure you're getting enough zinc.

A review of 32 studies published by the American Society for Nutrition found zinc supplements were linked to lower fasting blood sugar levels in people who had diabetes or were at a high risk of developing the disease. Experts think that zinc protects you by helping your body make and use insulin properly.

Researchers say more studies are needed to find out just how much zinc can help ward off or manage diabetes. In the meantime, you can stick with expert recommended doses. Men should aim for 11 milligrams (mg) of zinc every day while women need 8 mg. A single cup of cooked lentils clocks in with 2.5 mg.

Pass on gas: How to dodge this common discomfort

"I love beans, but they don't like me." Have you been known to say that, too? Beans are good for you, so don't avoid them because of the intestinal discomfort they can cause. To get all the nourishing benefits without any gassy side effects, follow these tips.

- Soak the dried beans for about four or five hours, then drain.

- Cover with fresh water and boil for 10 minutes. Simmer for 30 minutes.

- Drain and cover with more water. Simmer until the beans are tender, about one to two hours.

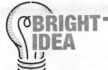

Bored with beans? Jazz up your dinner with a few simple twists

Let's face it. Tucking into a tired can of beans for your protein fix can get boring. Fortunately, you can easily bring those bland beans to life with these tasty tips.

- Blend 'em into a spread. Next time you make beans, combine them with a bit of lemon juice, olive oil, and your favorite herbs. Blend or mash them together until they're thick and spreadable. This puree is great on sandwiches, toast, or even served with chips.

- Make a healthy, zesty salad dressing. Rinse and drain half a can of white beans. Add them to a blender with 1 tablespoon of olive oil, 2 tablespoons of yogurt, a squirt of lemon juice and some herbs. Pulse until you have a creamy dressing.

- Satisfy your crunch cravings with a healthy alternative. Instead of reaching for a bag of potato chips, try making crispy chickpeas instead. Drain and rinse a can of chickpeas, pat them dry, and drizzle with olive oil. Then roast in a 400-degree oven for about 20 minutes, or until they're nice and crispy. Try tossing them with smoked paprika or a pinch of your favorite spices when they come out of the oven.

- Jazz up your smoothies with a few beans. Beans can help you get a thick, creamy smoothie while adding tons of fiber and protein. Simply add 1/4 to 1/2 cup of rinsed, drained beans to your favorite smoothie ingredients before blending.

Light therapy

Catch some rays for a brighter brain

Have you heard of Nicéphore Niépce? He was a French inventor who figured out how to use sunlight to take photographs through a process he called heliography — helios from the Greek word for "sun" and graphein meaning "writing." His most famous picture, "View from the Window at Le Gras," is the oldest surviving camera photograph.

Early photography — just one of the amazing processes made possible by sunlight. But your body uses sunlight in amazing ways, too, like sharpening your brain and lowering your blood pressure.

Time in the sun leads to cognitive clout. Researchers studied nearly 1,200 folks who were more than 59 years old and living in rural China to find out if sunshine had anything to do with cognitive abilities. They questioned the seniors about the amount of time they spent in the sun before the age of 60, and the time of day they were usually outside.

The people who had the most sun exposure spent three hours in the morning outside, and three more hours in the afternoon. Those with the least exposure spent two hours in the sun during the early morning and two in the late afternoon when the sun was lower. When it came to the cognitive abilities test, who do you suppose came out on top? Those with the most sunlight exposure.

Researchers believe it has to do with vitamin D, a nutrient made in your skin when it's exposed to the sun. High levels of vitamin D are thought to contribute to improved brain function.

Shine a light on better blood pressure. In a three-year study of more than 342,000 people on dialysis, researchers found that a sunny day does more than just lift sagging spirits. It may help lower your blood pressure, too. High blood pressure can cause blood clots in the arteries that lead to your brain, possibly bringing on a stroke. And narrowed or blocked arteries could also limit blood flow, leading to vascular dementia.

Nitric oxide (NO) is the real hero. It's a molecule whose most important function is to relax the inner muscles of your blood vessels, causing them to expand and increase your circulation.

> Hippocrates, the father of medicine, believed that cities properly oriented toward the sun would have less disease. Nurse Florence Nightingale must have agreed because she was a big supporter of letting as much natural light into her patients' rooms as possible. Research confirms sunlight has positive effects on human health. Let the sun shine in!

Roomier blood vessels lower your blood pressure, and that's good for your brain. Your skin stores lots of nitric oxide, which reacts to the sun's rays and hops into action when you head outside.

Worried about damaging rays and your skin? Talk to your doctor to balance those concerns against the blood pressure benefits of sunlight.

Light therapy flips the switch on depression and insomnia

From Edison's very first lightbulb to Darth Vader's deadly lightsaber, people have been intrigued by the power of light. After all, light is necessary for growing food and warming the planet. But researchers know that light can help in other ways, too. Even the artificial kind. Find out how modern light therapy can help with seasonal affective disorder, major depression, and sleep.

BLT blocks SAD. Changes in weather got you down in the dumps? People often use bright light therapy (BLT) to treat seasonal affective disorder (SAD), a kind of depression that may occur when folks face shorter days and less sunlight during the fall and winter.

Most people with SAD feel better after being exposed to bright light therapy — a treatment using artificial light that's brighter than indoor light but not as bright as direct sunlight. Ultraviolet light, full-spectrum light, heat lamps, and tanning lamps won't provide the same results.

Studies show bright light therapy works because it supplies the rays you're missing. And some researchers think the light triggers the production of the feel-good brain chemical serotonin.

Think inside the box to ease depression. Basking in the glow of a light box may also help other forms of depression. For example, researchers conducted an eight-week study of light therapy's effects on 122 adults, ages 19 through 60. Doctors had diagnosed each person in the study with major depressive disorder.

The participants were divided into four groups. The groups received only light therapy, only medication, a combination of both, or neither. Researchers saw the biggest drop in depression scores in the group that received both light therapy and medication.

Turn on a light to get some sleep. If you suffer from insomnia, you probably know what an exhausted brain feels like. Maybe you can't concentrate, or you're struggling with memory loss and mood swings. A sleep-deprived brain is associated with an increased risk for depression, hallucinations, and impulsive behavior.

But a meta-analysis of 53 studies shows that light therapy improves sleep problems, including those related to dementia and insomnia. Exposure to bright light can help you get better sleep by adjusting your body's circadian rhythm — your inner clock that tells your body when to be awake and when to be asleep.

Take home the right box of sunshine

In the market for a light box of your own? From a lamp you can place on your desk to a visor you wear on your head, you'll find many different styles — and prices. Here are a few things to consider before you choose.

Your doctor might be able to tell you which light boxes his patients prefer as well as which ones to stay away from. If you've had eye problems related to cataracts, glaucoma, or diabetes, talk to your eye doctor about the risks of using a light box.

Prices for light boxes range from around $30 to close to $300 online. And since light boxes haven't been approved by the Food and Drug Administration, many insurance plans won't pay for them. Luckily, a less expensive box — one without all the bells and whistles — may offer everything you need.

Your box should provide you with exposure to at least 10,000 lux of light. And you want it to give off as little ultraviolet (UV) light as possible to avoid hurting your eyes.

Your light box should be convenient to use and easy to set up in the right location. For example, your family room may accommodate a large box, while your office is better suited for a small, desk-lamp style. Be sure to check the manufacturer's directions so you get the right amount of light at the right distance.

Low-fat diet

Eat smart to dodge dementia

Fats sure have gotten a bad rap over the years. But they're an important part of your diet. For example, the healthy fats found in nuts, avocados, salmon, and tuna are good for your heart. But the kind of unhealthy fats in fast food, processed meats, and pastries have the opposite effect. Not only do they increase your risk of heart disease and stroke, they put you on the fast track to dementia.

You need some fat in your diet. It's just a matter of choosing the right kind and the right amount.

Want to sidestep dementia? Steer clear of saturated fats. You know all those fats that are solid at room temperature — like butter, lard, and coconut oil? Experts say you should avoid them if you want to keep your brain healthy. They're known as saturated fats, and new research suggests they may lead to dementia and Alzheimer's.

A recent review published in *Current Alzheimer's Research* looked at four studies that linked fat intake to cognitive decline. Researchers concluded a diet high in saturated fat more than doubled participants' risk of developing dementia. And Alzheimer's disease? Lots of saturated fats increased their risk of developing the disease by 39%.

The American Heart Association recommends keeping your saturated fat intake below 13 grams a day. The organization suggests swapping fatty red meat for lean meats, poultry, beans, and legumes. Another option? Use olive oil instead of butter.

Follow a low-fat diet to stave off cognitive decline. Need another reason to cut back on bad fats? Recent research reveals that a low-fat diet can slash your risk of age-related cognitive impairment.

Scientists divided 1,606 senior women into two groups. Some stuck with their normal diets. Others were told to increase the amount of fruits, vegetables, and grains they ate while cutting the amount of fat in their diets to no more than 20% of their calories. So if they ate 2,000 calories in a day, they could only have 44 grams of fat.

The researchers tested the cognitive function of the women annually over 8 1/2 years. They found that those who followed the low-fat diet were significantly less likely to develop age-related cognitive impairment.

Experts think this diet works because it helps reduce major risk factors of dementia, including diabetes and hypertension.

Triple threat — tackle this trio with a low-fat diet

It's sad but true — some 7 in 10 Americans are overweight or obese. And when it comes to carrying around extra weight, the strain on your joints is just the tip of the iceberg. Too much body fat puts you at risk for heart disease and diabetes, serious conditions that increase your chances of developing dementia.

The good news? A low-fat diet can help you steer clear of these dangerous health issues.

Cut down on fat to ward off heart disease and diabetes. Heart disease and diabetes often go hand in hand. That's because high blood sugar damages the blood vessels and nerves that control your heart. Fortunately, research suggests that eating less fat can help keep both diseases at bay.

In a large-scale study published in *The Journal of Nutrition*, researchers recruited nearly 49,000 women between the ages of 50 and 79 and asked them to follow either a low-fat diet or to stick to their normal meal plans.

A long-term follow-up found that the women who reduced the fat in their diet significantly lowered their risk of type 1 diabetes and coronary heart disease (CHD). CHD develops when a buildup of plaque narrows your arteries and prevents them from delivering enough blood to your heart.

The women on the low-fat diet cut their fat intake to about 20% of their daily calories, which is the low end of what experts recommended. And they didn't only cut back on fat. They replaced those calories with fruit, veggies, and healthy grains.

Need a new diet? Melt pounds away with the low-fat plan. In the early 1900s, an art dealer named Horace Fletcher became famous for developing the Chewing Diet. The premise was simple — chew each bite of food at least 32 times and then spit it out. While there's no scientific data that says this absurd practice will help you lose weight, experts have the data to back up the effectiveness of the low-fat diet.

Researchers asked 609 overweight adults to follow either a healthy low-fat or a healthy low-carb diet for one year. Afterward, researchers checked in with the two groups and found both diets to be equally effective. Participants on the low-fat diet lost an average of 11.7 pounds. And those on the low-carb diet? 13.2 pounds. That's why experts say you should pick the diet you'll stick with in the long run.

> Healthy fats help your body transport and absorb vitamins. That's why you need to include unsaturated fat in your diet. Opt for fats that are liquid at room temperature — like olive, flaxseed, sunflower, canola, and peanut oils.

So why is a low-fat diet so effective? When you swap fats for foods with more fiber and water, you feel fuller longer and aren't tempted to overeat.

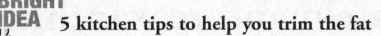

5 kitchen tips to help you trim the fat

Want to cut down on fat without compromising on flavor? With a little know-how in your kitchen, you can create delicious low-fat meals.

- Make smart swaps for better baking. Does a recipe call for butter or oil? You can use the same amount of low-fat yogurt or even sugar-free applesauce to keep your baked goods moist, flavorful, and healthy.

- Spice up your meals with low-fat substitutes. Don't drench your salad with fatty dressings. And stop seasoning your veggies with butter and oil. Instead, ramp up the flavor with a sprinkling of spices or a splash of lemon juice.

- Cut out the cooking fat. Sauteing and deep frying your food adds extra fat to your dinner plate. Instead, consider steaming, poaching, or roasting your meats, veggies, and fish so that you don't have to add any oil or butter. If you want to fry in a pan, use a small spritz of nonstick vegetable oil spray.

- Get creative with your mix-ins. Family favorites like hamburgers and meatloaf are often high in fat. Instead of changing the menu entirely, mix ground meat with mushrooms, cooked lentils, or cooked beans. You'll cut down on the fat and still have a dinner that tastes rich and meaty.

- Skim excess grease. When you're making a soup or a stew, you might notice little beads of fat forming on the top. Simply take a spoon or a ladle and scoop off any extra fat.

Lutein and zeaxanthin

Can color change your mind? In your food, maybe so

Media hype would have you believe that restaurant chains use a calculated color strategy — a so-called Ketchup and Mustard theory — to make you hungry and lure you in. Maybe red and yellow logos sway your behavior in restaurants, or maybe they don't. Regardless, nutrition experts have good evidence to tell you to eat red, yellow, orange, and green foods.

In fact, colors are a clue that these delicious foods contain a powerful nutrient called lutein that can boost your memory and protect your brain.

This carotenoid, or pigment, not only gives some fruits and veggies their vibrant hues, but it also hangs out in your brain where it offers mind-blowing benefits. For example, in at least one large study of seniors, researchers found that higher levels of lutein could decrease the risk of Alzheimer's disease.

All in all, the nutrient has more to offer your brain than you might expect.

Make memories with your berries. Botanists agree. The avocado is a berry. And this berry adds lutein to your diet. So why not put it on your grocery list? A study funded by the Haas Avocado Board found that one avocado a day for six months improved performance on working memory and problem-solving tasks.

Unsurprisingly, the researchers chalk it up to the lutein. To get more of this nutrient, you can also try avocado's berry cousins, papaya and kiwi. Or fill up on carrots, sweet potatoes, and spinach. Your noggin will thank you, particularly the part involved in memory and learning — the hippocampus.

That's what researchers discovered in a separate study recently published in *Nutrients*. They chose a group of overweight and obese adults and measured the level of lutein in their blood after fasting overnight.

Participants also completed tasks that tested their relational memory, a hippocampus-dependent ability to remember associations between objects and events. That's the kind of memory you use to retell a story of a road trip in any order or name someone you've seen before. Researchers found higher blood levels of lutein predicted better performance on the memory tests.

Lutein levels the playing field for older brains. Does lutein up your brain game? It's possible, according to researchers at the University of Illinois. They measured the carotenoid level in the retina of the eye, since amounts there correlate with lutein levels in the brain.

Participants then took three attention tests while researchers measured neural activity in their brains. Results showed middle-aged participants with higher lutein levels had neural responses that were more on par with younger people than with folks their age who had lower lutein concentrations.

"Now there's an additional reason to eat nutrient-rich foods such as green leafy vegetables, eggs, and avocados," says Naiman Khan, a professor of kinesiology and community health at Illinois. "We know these foods are related to other health benefits, but these data indicate that there may be cognitive benefits as well."

A feast for your eyes may protect your vision

Imagine you're admiring a paper copy of a favorite family photo. You take a sip of iced tea and a droplet falls from your glass onto the center of the picture. The faces smudge — now unrecognizable — leaving the rest unharmed.

Everything may look like that blurred photo for someone with age-related macular degeneration (AMD). The macula in the back of the eye becomes damaged, so you find it harder to see fine details in the center of your vision — just like in the blurred picture.

Fortunately, you can feed your eyes nutrients like lutein and zeaxanthin that may protect you against AMD.

Want to see into the future? Take care of your macula. Since your macula helps you see central details, it's vital for activities like driving, recognizing faces, and using a computer. Although small, this powerful yellow oval in your retina also absorbs harmful light rays to protect cells in your eye from damage.

Your macula is packed with lutein and zeaxanthin — carotenoids responsible for that yellow color. When you don't have enough lutein and zeaxanthin, you are at a greater risk for AMD. Unfortunately, AMD is a leading cause of vision loss for people over 55.

But there's good news. Current evidence suggests that getting more lutein and zeaxanthin from the foods you eat can play an important role in protecting you against AMD, especially if you are at a higher risk.

Tantalizing tips to get more lutein and zeaxanthin. Liven up your lunches or dress out your dinners with more foods that have these nutrients. But when you're writing up your grocery list, keep in mind some food combos actually help you get more eye-supporting carotenoids. Cue the fat.

When you add fat in the form of foods that already contain lutein and zeaxanthin — eggs or pistachio nuts, for example — you improve your chances of absorbing more of the good stuff. Or break out the olive oil to sautee your leafy greens and red or green peppers. You might even drizzle some almonds with oil and toast them in the oven.

Not getting enough lutein and zeaxanthin the natural way? Supplements may be a good option for you. They were linked to sharper vision for people with AMD in a meta-analysis of seven studies. And you get a bonus — lutein supplements have been associated with higher scores on verbal fluency tests.

The bottom line? Eating foods loaded with lutein and zeaxanthin could protect your eyes. And that helps your brain, too. New research links poor vision with an increased risk of developing cognitive decline.

Sight stealers — the surprising source of peeper problems

Vision trouble? It might not have anything to do with your lutein and zeaxanthin levels. Some eye issues come from a surprising source — medications.

Cloudy, burning, scratchy, itchy, or pink eyes aren't normal. Take a look at the possible side effects of medications you may be using.

- cataracts — cholesterol meds like atorvastatin or lovastatin, and corticosteroids like prednisone

- double, blurred, or altered vision — antidepressants, alpha-blockers like alfuzosin, cholesterol meds, erectile dysfunction drugs like sildenafil, osteoporosis meds like alendronate, and antibiotics

- eye infections — corticosteroids and osteoporosis meds

- glaucoma — antihistamines, epilepsy and migraine meds like topiramate, and diuretics for high blood pressure

- dry eye — antidepressants and anxiety meds

- light sensitivity or pain — alpha-blockers, erectile dysfunction drugs, and osteoporosis meds

Call your doctor to schedule an appointment right away if you notice any changes with your eyes. Be sure to take a list of your medications with you.

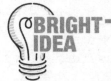

Build a better meal for your brain and baby blues

Even if you don't have lutein and zeaxanthin on your mind, your brain and your eyes still need them. Experts don't yet have a fixed daily amount for these two pigments. But based on several eye studies, they do suggest loading your plate with fruits and veggies to get close to 10 milligrams (mg) of lutein and 2 mg of zeaxanthin a day.

Check out some of these top performers when it comes to supplying your lutein and zeaxanthin (L&Z) needs.

Food	Amount	Milligrams of L&Z
kale, cooked with oil	1 cup	23.60
spinach, cooked with oil	1 cup	19.70
collards, cooked with oil	1 cup	8.01
squash or zucchini, raw	1 medium	4.16
parsley, fresh, chopped	1 cup	3.34
fennel, cooked with oil	1 bulb	1.82
persimmon	1 fruit	1.40
asparagus, raw	1 cup	0.95
avocado, mashed	1 cup	0.62
green pepper, cooked with oil	1 medium	0.49
artichoke, cooked in oil	1 small globe	0.46
basil leaves, fresh	1/4 cup	0.34
egg, fried	1 large	0.25
cayenne pepper	1 teaspoon	0.24
red cabbage, raw, chopped	1 cup	0.29
papaya	1 small	0.14
peaches, sliced	1 cup	0.14
apricots, halved	1 cup	0.14
blueberries	1 cup	0.12

Lycopene

Think better, feel better with one nutrient

Never heard of lycopene? No worries. It's a plant pigment, called a carotenoid, that gives many red and pink fruits their characteristic colors. What's more, lycopene is a powerful nutrient capable of keeping your thoughts on track and depression at bay.

Work smarter, not harder, with lycopene. The key to better brain health is in your blood. That's according to researchers who found that nutrients running through your veins, including lycopene, are linked to better brain function.

Researchers measured the nutrients in the blood of more than 100 healthy seniors. They discovered that the volunteers who had higher levels of lycopene — along with omega-3 and omega-6 fatty acids, carotenoids, vitamin D, and various B vitamins — performed better on cognitive tests.

In addition to memory, those tests measured both general intelligence and executive function — the skills you need to follow directions, control your emotions, and focus.

The scientists believe the nutrients work collectively to keep aging brains in tiptop shape.

This antioxidant mends your mood. Scientists believe unstable atoms called free radicals may play a role in the development of mental health conditions like depression. That's why they think eating your fill of fruits and vegetables packed with antioxidants — molecules that give those dangerous free radicals a run for their money — may be key to fighting the blues.

Lycopene, it turns out, is the most powerful antioxidant among the carotenoids. And because tomatoes are a major source of lycopene, researchers turned to this mighty fruit to study its relationship to depression.

In a Japanese study, nearly 1,000 people age 70 and older were surveyed about their diet and symptoms of depression. The scientists found that the seniors who ate tomatoes two to six times a week were 46% less likely to report mild or severe depressive symptoms compared with those who ate tomatoes less than once a week.

Even more astounding, those who ate tomatoes once or more a day were 52% less likely to have symptoms of depression than the other group. "These results suggest that a tomato-rich diet may have a beneficial effect on the prevention of depressive symptoms," the researchers concluded.

5 foods that give you a lycopene lift

Unlike other nutrients, there isn't an established daily recommended amount of lycopene. But Dr. Edward Giovannucci, a professor of nutrition and epidemiology at the Harvard School of Public Health, recommends getting at least 10,000 micrograms (mcg) of lycopene per day.

That may sound like a lot, but it's easier than you think. The following foods offer a variety of flavors along with high amounts of lycopene.

Food	Lycopene (mcg) per cup
tomato juice, canned	21,960
guava	8,587
tomatoes, cooked	7,298
papaya	2,651
grapefruit	2,610

Take a bite out of bad health with lycopene

Did you know that tomatoes aren't vegetables? They're fruits. Specifically, berries. Here's something else interesting about tomatoes. They're jam packed with lycopene, a natural chemical that can lower bad cholesterol levels and help fight inflammation of the gums.

Call off a cholesterol crisis with this nutrient. Too much cholesterol can block the arteries leading to your brain, increasing your risk of developing dementia. But new research published in *Nutrients* shows that tomatoes abundant in lycopene can reduce the LDL cholesterol — the bad kind of cholesterol — that builds up in the walls of your arteries.

The study used a tomato specially bred to have above-normal amounts of lycopene. About half of the 74 participants ate a little less than 2 ounces of this tomato daily over three months. The rest were given the same amount of tomato modified to have no lycopene. When the 12 weeks were up, the people who ate the lycopene-rich tomatoes saw significant improvements in their LDL cholesterol levels compared with the placebo group.

Adding this juicy fruit to your diet is a simple change you can make to help lower bad cholesterol levels and reduce your risk of coronary heart disease.

> Some 80% of the lycopene in the American diet comes from tomatoes. But not all tomatoes have the same amount of lycopene. According to one study, raw cherry and roma tomatoes provide optimal amounts of this much-needed carotenoid. Vine tomatoes? Not as much.

Lycopene doles out dental help. You may have gingivitis if your gums are puffy and bleed easily. Left untreated, gingivitis can cause tooth loss and other serious health complications — including dementia. Scientists have found that bacteria in your mouth are able to move to your brain and release enzymes that destroy nerve cells. That could lead to memory loss and Alzheimer's disease.

Research suggests that diets low in antioxidants — compounds that prevent or slow damage to your cells — may make you more susceptible to gingivitis and other unhealthy oral conditions. That's why scientists believe you may be able to protect your gums and teeth with the food you eat.

One study found that lycopene can be an important part of your dental care. Sixty healthy adults with mild gingivitis were divided into two groups. Both underwent a deep-cleaning process called scaling and root planing. But only half of the participants also took an antioxidant supplement containing lycopene, turmeric, and piperine twice a day for three weeks.

Not surprisingly, both groups showed a reduction in gingivitis symptoms. But the volunteers who took the supplement experienced greater improvements — including lower amounts of plaque and less inflammation — than the control group. According to the researchers, the anti-inflammatory and antioxidant effects of this supplement suggest that lycopene can help fight gingivitis.

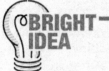

BRIGHT IDEA

Recipe for success: 4 ways to jazz up your tomato juice

Not wild about the taste of tomato juice? If so, you're missing out on a particularly rich source of lycopene. Try these flavor fixes to make your juice journey more enjoyable. If you're already a fan, use them as inspiration for your next tasty concoction.

- Sweet. Mix apple, carrot, or grape juice with tomato juice to step up your flavor and nutrition profile. One part fruit juice to three parts tomato juice should do the trick.

- Spicy. Liven up your drink with classic hot sauce. Pour 1 1/2 teaspoons of Tabasco or Worcestershire sauce into a quart of tomato juice.

- Savory. If you're looking for a deeper flavor without the spicy kick, try a pinch of herbs. Coriander, pepper, and cumin all make mouthwatering options.

- Fresh. Add garden freshness to your drink with celery and onion for a veggie-packed taste.

Magnesium

Mind the nutrition gap — this mighty mineral sustains your brain

"When placed in command, take charge." Those were the wise words of "Stormin' Norman" Schwarzkopf, the late four-star general who commanded allied troops in the 1991 Gulf War. True not only for the well-being of his soldiers, but for anyone in the heat of battle. Like you.

You're sparring every day to stay healthy in your senior years. Could a simple mineral deficiency be causing the symptoms you're fighting? Find out what you need to be eating to stop fatigue, leg cramps, headaches, brain fog, mood swings, and more. After all, you're in command of your health. Time to take charge.

Magnesium battles brain complaints. Research shows that magnesium levels in people with Alzheimer's disease (AD) are lower than normal. In fact, low magnesium in certain parts of the brain may be a factor in developing AD, the most common form of dementia.

So to find out more, researchers conducted an eight-year study of more than 1,400 healthy older adults. They followed the participants' diets by asking them questions about 215 food items, including cooking methods, serving sizes, eating habits, and the use of supplements. The scientists used the responses to estimate the participants' magnesium intake.

At the end of the study, researchers found that the volunteers with higher levels of magnesium in their diet had a decreased risk of mild cognitive impairment (MCI). MCI is the stage between the expected decline in memory and thinking that comes with aging and the more serious decline of dementia. Your best bet? Up your magnesium to knock down your risk of developing dementia.

Combatting depression? Partner with a winner. A study of 112 adults with mild to moderate depression tested the effectiveness and safety of over-the-counter magnesium for treating depression. Participants took 248 milligrams (mg) of magnesium daily for six weeks. At the end of the study, the researchers found that the volunteers' depression and anxiety symptoms showed significant improvement compared with a six-week period in which they didn't take the supplement.

Researchers aren't sure why magnesium helps people with depression. But they know that magnesium plays an important role in regulating your mood. And if you don't have enough magnesium in your body, high levels of calcium and the neurotransmitter glutamate may band together to hinder the communication between nerve cells in your brain. That can lead to depression.

The final word? Make sure you get enough magnesium every day to decrease your depression and anxiety symptoms.

Add these delicious foods to your arsenal. Men age 30 and older should try to get 420 mg of magnesium every day. Women in the same age bracket should aim for 320 mg. Try these magnesium-packed favorites to get the support you need.

- nuts and seeds like almonds, cashews, and pumpkin seeds

- legumes like beans and peanuts

- fruits like pineapple, bananas, and figs

- vegetables like spinach and okra

- grains like brown rice

> No pricey bath bombs needed for this spa-like experience. Just add 1 1/2 cups of good old-fashioned Epsom salts — also known as magnesium sulfate — to a bathtub of hot water. Relax as your stress, anxiety, and muscle aches float away. Be sure to buy 100% magnesium sulfate. It's the best quality.

Keep in top-notch condition with this nourishing nutrient

A pounding heart and weak knees — sure signs you're falling in love? Well, maybe. But it's more likely you need to have your doctor monitor your magnesium, the heart-helping, bone-bettering must-have mineral.

For a positive change of heart, go with magnesium. Suppose you could reduce your risk of stroke by adding one simple nutrient to your diet. Would you do it? Of course you would. A review of several studies found that people who had higher amounts of magnesium in their diets ran a lower risk of having a stroke. In fact, the risk for an ischemic stroke — the kind of stroke that occurs when a clot blocks a blood vessel in the brain — fell by 9% for each additional 100 milligrams (mg) of magnesium participants ate each day.

Looking to boost your magnesium? An ounce of dry roasted almonds or a cup of cooked brown rice will give you 80 mg. A cup of boiled black beans, meanwhile, provides 120 mg. And a cup of cooked spinach? A whopping 157 mg. Researchers think magnesium lowers your stroke risk by stabilizing your heart rhythms. In addition, the mineral has anti-inflammatory and anti-clotting properties.

Turn down the pressure with one simple supplement. Another way magnesium keeps you healthy is by regulating your blood pressure. A review of 34 studies of more than 2,000 adults found that those who took magnesium supplements had lower blood pressure after three months compared with those who didn't take supplements.

Researchers think magnesium helps keep your blood vessels relaxed, which allows for increased blood flow and prevents rises in blood pressure that can lead to heart and brain damage.

This mineral rocks you to the bone. And to the muscle, too. Researchers checked the grip strength, skeletal muscle strength, and bone mineral density of nearly 157,000 men and women between the ages of 39 and 72 to learn if magnesium could help prevent osteoporosis and sarcopenia. Osteoporosis is a condition in which your bones become weak and brittle. Sarcopenia is the loss of muscle mass and function. And both have been linked to dementia.

The participants' intake of magnesium was determined by a question-naire. The results showed that those with higher intakes of magnesium had better grip strength, bone mineral density, and skeletal muscle mass than those with lower intakes. To sum up, the researchers determined that magnesium — along with protein and calcium — has an important role in keeping your muscles and bones strong.

BRIGHT IDEA

All out of leafy greens?
These supplements fill the magnesium gap

Your doctor probably told you it's best to get the magnesium you need through your food every day. But sometimes that's tough to do. If you have a magnesium deficiency, ask your physician if it's safe for you to use one of the supplements below.

- Magnesium lactate supports your nervous system, heart, and digestive system. It's also used to treat indigestion.

- Magnesium taurate may be just what you need to protect your heart and control high blood sugar.

- Magnesium oxide relieves heartburn and constipation.

- Magnesium glycinate may help reduce depression and insomnia.

- Magnesium chloride eases heartburn and adjusts magnesium levels.

- Magnesium orotate is linked to improved energy production in heart tissue.

- Magnesium L-threonate may help manage depression and memory loss.

- Magnesium citrate is used to raise magnesium levels and treat constipation.

- Magnesium malate may reduce fatigue and muscle pain.

Massage therapy

Soothe stress, anxiety, and depression with this relaxing treatment

Think of massages as an occasional indulgence? Well, you don't need to be on vacation to reap the benefits of massage therapy. Medical experts say you have a good reason to make this soothing treatment a regular part of your routine.

A recent review published in *Focus* examined multiple studies about massage therapy and its role in improving your mood. Experts think getting a massage, especially alongside other treatments, can help fight off anxiety and depression. The research is early, though, so more studies need to be done.

Still, scientists have a theory as to why taking a trip to the spa can lift your spirits. People with depression often have more brain activity in their right frontal lobe. And this is associated with negative emotions and withdrawal behaviors.

After a short session of moderate-pressure massage, brain activity in depressed adults has shifted from the right to the left. Even better? Chemical compounds in the brain that spike when you're feeling blue have gone down following these massages. In addition, the feel-good chemicals serotonin and dopamine have increased.

Still on the fence about massage therapy? It might be intimidating if you've never done it before. So instead of going all in, consider a head massage. It may help you soothe stress and feel refreshed without committing to a full body massage.

A hands-on approach rubs away this painful duo

Chinese and Indian healers have been using massages for thousands of years. They claim this ancient practice can cure disease, soothe pain, and even prevent illness. And now researchers say massage therapy might live up to some of these promises.

Need a knee up on OA? Try a massage. You might only think about getting a massage when your muscles are tight. But new research suggests this treatment can soothe arthritis flare-ups, too.

In a new study, 200 people with knee osteoarthritis (OA) received hourlong weekly Swedish massages, light-touch therapy, or no treatment. After eight weeks, the massage group reported lower levels of pain and stiffness than the other groups.

Scientists think the improvements were due to reduced inflammation from the massages. And that's great news for your joints and your brain. A recent analysis showed an association between OA and an increased risk of dementia. Researchers say the link could be due to harmful molecules called cytokines that promote inflammation.

Say goodbye to migraines with a simple massage. Migraine sufferers know all too well that these headaches can cause brain fog. It's impossible to concentrate on the simplest task when you're under attack from a migraine. Fortunately, regular massages may help keep those symptoms at bay.

And a specific type — known as a lymphatic drainage massage — may be the most effective. This treatment targets your lymph nodes, which help filter foreign cells and bacteria from your body.

Researchers recruited 64 women with frequent migraines and split them up into three groups. Some got a 30-minute traditional massage or lymphatic drainage massage once a week for eight weeks. The third group didn't get any treatment. The women also recorded how often they got migraines.

After the study was over, the researchers found that both massages helped cut down on the frequency of migraines compared to the control group. What's more, women who got lymphatic drainage massages needed less over-the-counter painkillers.

Talk to your doctor to see if this technique could be right for you. If you have congestive heart failure, an infection in your lymphatic system, or a high risk of blood clotting, lymphatic drainage massages could pose a risk to your health.

BRIGHT IDEA

Learn to make the most of your massage

Not sure where to start? You've probably seen massage chairs at the mall or the airport, but if you want to get all the healing benefits you'll need to track down the real deal and prepare for your first appointment.

- Pick the right therapist. If you need a therapeutic massage, chances are you won't find it at a mall kiosk. Look for someone licensed by the state and professional organizations. They either have the title CMT (certified massage therapist) or LMT (licensed massage therapist). And ask if they have malpractice insurance. If they don't, it's a sign you should look elsewhere. You can ask your doctor, friends, or physical therapist for recommendations.

- Discuss your needs. Once you've picked out who will give you a massage, you need to decide on what you want. But if you don't know the difference between a Swedish and a shiatsu, talk to your therapist. She will help you identify the perfect treatment. Once the massage starts, speak up. Some techniques might cause slight discomfort, but if something is too intense or painful you need to tell the therapist at once.

- Stay in your comfort zone. Massages are all about you, so make sure you're comfortable. Let your therapist know if you'd rather remain clothed during your massage. And don't be shy if the room is too hot or too cold, or if you just don't like the music that's playing.

Mediterranean diet

Want to triple your brain defense? Try this delightful diet

Researchers in the 1960s noticed that people from Mediterranean countries often had lower rates of heart disease. Eventually, they realized the region's diets — which are rich in olive oil, fruits, leafy greens, fatty fish, and other nutritional powerhouses — help fight off other chronic conditions, too. Now scientists think you may protect your brain by following the same delicious diet.

Want to slow the progress of Alzheimer's? Take your meals to the Mediterranean. Experts say preventing cognitive decline could begin with your dinner plate. If you start following the Mediterranean diet now you may keep your brain sharp, even if you're a senior.

Researchers scanned the brains of adults between the ages of 30 and 60 who either followed a Western-style diet or ate mostly Mediterranean meals. At least two years later, they followed up with the participants and looked at their brains again.

People who followed a Western-style diet had more beta-amyloid deposits in their brains than those on the Mediterranean diet. Researchers say those deposits are early markers of dementia. And they estimate sticking to a Mediterranean diet long term may offer up to 3 1/2 years of protection against brain aging and Alzheimer's.

One possible reason is this diet limits foods that are known to cause heart disease, insulin resistance, and inflammation — which could all speed up brain aging.

Eat smarter to steer clear of a shrinking brain. The Mediterranean diet helps you load up on fruits, veggies, fish, and nuts, and encourages you to cut down on sugar. And that's important if you want to keep your mind in tiptop shape. As you get older, your brain shrinks in areas associated with memory and learning, which can affect mental function. But a better diet is linked to a bigger brain.

In a recent study, researchers asked 4,213 seniors to fill out questionnaires detailing everything they ate in an average month. Then they scanned the participants' heads to see if the foods they favored had an impact on their brains. Surprisingly, the people who drank fewer sugary drinks and ate more healthy foods — like fruit, veggies, fish, nuts, whole grains, and dairy — had more gray and white brain matter. Plus they had bigger hippocampi — the region of the brain responsible for storing memories.

Beat the blues with the Mediterranean diet. Taking a vacation to the Mediterranean sea would be a great way to lift your mood. But if you can't spend all your days in sunny Spain, you can still bring some of the mood-boosting benefits of the Mediterranean back home.

A small study, published in *Nutrients*, asked people at risk for cardiovascular disease to follow a Mediterranean diet with lean pork or a low-fat diet for eight weeks. Then participants took a two-month break before swapping diets and repeating the experiment.

While people were following the Mediterranean diet, they had higher scores on surveys measuring emotional role functioning, which involves issues experienced in daily life due to anxiety and depression. The researchers think the diet may help by fighting inflammation, which is linked to the development of depression.

New research suggests a Mediterranean diet may protect seniors from more than heart disease and dementia. The fiber, vitamins, and minerals in this diet help boost the bacteria in your gut that are linked with healthy aging, reduced frailty, and lower levels of inflammation.

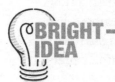

Set the table with these 3 simple Mediterranean meals

Scientists say the Mediterranean diet can work like medicine against heart disease, diabetes, arthritis, dementia, vision loss, and even sleep problems. Need a bit of advice on getting more of these foods in your diet? This daily menu calls on 12 Mediterranean staples to make healthy meals.

Start your day with barley porridge. You might only think of oatmeal when you want a hot bowl of porridge. But other whole grains are great choices, too.

Simmer 3/4 cup of pearled barley with 4 cups of water or milk for 45 minutes, until it's thick and creamy. Top it with sliced bananas, chopped prunes, raisins, and your favorite nuts for a sweet way to start the day.

Amp up your salad for a better lunch. Want a midday meal that won't leave your stomach rumbling an hour later? Simply toss spinach with a handful of cooked lentils and a few sardines.

Serve it alongside a simple dressing made by mixing together plain yogurt, a splash of lemon juice, and a handful of your favorite herbs.

Spice up your dinner with a quinoa and broccoli curry.
In a medium pot, simmer 1/2 cup of quinoa in 1 cup of water for 15 minutes, or until tender. Remove from the pot and fluff with a fork.

Then add chopped broccoli, onions, ginger, and garlic to the pot and cook on medium heat until tender. Sprinkle in 2 teaspoons of curry powder and stir the quinoa back in. Pair it with a baked salmon filet for a complete dinner.

6 ways a Mediterranean menu keeps your vision sharp for years

Fading eyesight is bad news for your brain. A recent study shows that losing your vision is associated with faster cognitive decline. Fortunately, revitalizing your aging eyes is easy with the right foods. The Mediterranean diet can help you get all the nutrients your eyes need to fend off glaucoma, cataracts, age-related macular degeneration (AMD), and night blindness.

Fatty fish. Tuna, salmon, and sardines are loaded with omega-3 fatty acids. And researchers say these healthy fats may protect your eyesight. A study published in *The American Journal of Clinical Nutrition* found that people who ate fatty fish at least once a week halved their risk of AMD compared with those who ate fish less often.

Leafy greens. Don't want to lose your precious vision to macular degeneration? Leafy green veggies are loaded with lutein and zeaxanthin, two protective nutrients that can keep your eyesight sharp for years to come. A single cup of raw spinach weighs in with a hefty 3.66 milligrams (mg) of this dynamic duo.

Yellow veggies. If you don't get enough vitamin A, you're at risk for night blindness. Fortunately, stocking up on foods like carrots and yellow squash are a perfect way to get this vital vitamin. That's because the chemical that gives these veggies their color — beta carotene — turns into vitamin A in your body.

Citrus. Oranges and grapefruits could be nature's all-natural cataract preventers. Studies show that getting more vitamin C into your diet may lower the development of cataracts. A single grapefruit will get you more than 75 mg — the amount of vitamin C recommended daily for women.

But stick to vitamin C-rich foods. Long-term use of high-dose vitamin C supplements — more than 500 mg a day — can actually increase your risk of cataracts.

Beans, peas, and lentils. Legumes are a great source of niacin. And if you want to fend off cloudy vision, you can't beat this nutritional go-getter. Researchers examined the diets of 16,770 people. And they found that people who got more niacin were also at lower risk for glaucoma. You'll get 3 mg from a cup of peas to go toward the daily recommended 14 mg for women over age 50 and 16 mg for men over 50.

Nuts and seeds. The landmark Age-Related Eye Disease Study (AREDS) revealed zinc may help ward off advanced AMD in people at high risk. A follow-up to that study shows that an AREDS supplement combination of antioxidants and 25 mg of zinc can help those people, too. And nuts and seeds are great sources of zinc. A 1-ounce serving of pumpkin seeds has 2.1 mg.

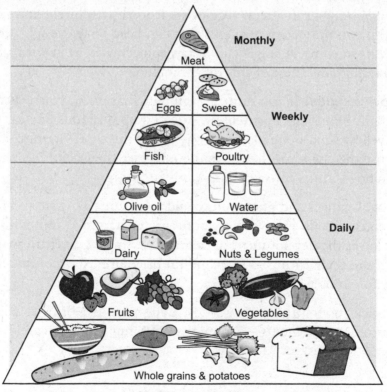

Mediterranean diet

Melatonin

Awaken to a better life — 2 ways this natural remedy protects your brain

"Hello darkness my old friend. I've come to talk with you again," crooned Paul Simon in the spring of 1964. Simon would later say he was giving voice to his "post-teenage angst." But his words also ring true for the millions of Americans who suffer from insomnia. It's a common problem among older folks, in part because the production of melatonin — a hormone that regulates the sleep-wake cycle — declines with age.

Unfortunately, low levels of melatonin have also been linked to a higher risk for Alzheimer's disease (AD) and migraines. But boosting the amount of this hormone in your body may help keep these conditions at bay.

Sleep soundly to fight AD. Did you know that sleep plays an important role in the consolidation of memories? It's essential for learning new things. So if you don't sleep well or can't doze off, you could be setting yourself up for a decline in cognitive performance.

But here's the good news. Melatonin may be able to restore your sleep cycle — and the sleep cycles of people with dementia — to normal. That's what scientists found when they tested the effects of the hormone on seniors who were taking medication to treat mild to moderate AD.

Eighty participants took either 2 milligrams (mg) of melatonin or a placebo one to two hours before bedtime for 24 weeks. By the end of the study, the melatonin group was able to sleep for longer lengths of time than the placebo group. They also performed better on tests measuring their cognitive function.

Consider the melatonin switch for migraine prevention. About half of the people who suffer from regular migraines stop seeking care for their headaches. One reason why? The side effects from prescription medicine. But research suggests these folks — who often have low levels of melatonin — may find relief by taking supplements.

Thinking about taking melatonin? Check with your doctor first. Melatonin can interact with your medications. Side effects can include daytime drowsiness and dizziness. And older people with dementia may metabolize melatonin more slowly. That could worsen daytime functioning.

Researchers asked 178 adults who experienced regular migraines to take one of three treatments at bedtime for 12 weeks. Participants were randomly assigned to take 3 mg of melatonin, a placebo, or 25 mg of amitriptyline, a drug sometimes prescribed to prevent migraines.

The results? Melatonin was just as effective as amitriptyline in preventing migraines. What's more, when compared with the amitriptyline group, those who took melatonin experienced these additional benefits.

- a greater reduction in the time spent with headaches
- a higher rate of having their migraine frequency cut in half
- fewer side effects

Dare to dream of better sleep and a slimmer waistline

In the habit of watching TV to wind down at bedtime? You may be trading precious melatonin for a dose of sleep-defying blue light. That's right. Your TV screen emits blue light — short wavelengths visible to the naked eye — that can block your production of melatonin.

That's why experts recommend you cut off electronic gadgets two to three hours before bedtime.

Here's another tip. Getting enough melatonin in your diet may ensure a good night's sleep and help keep your weight in check.

Reset your circadian rhythm for sounder sleep. Waking up with the daylight and falling asleep in the dark is part of your body's natural circadian rhythm. If this internal clock is off or your melatonin is low, your sleep cycle and ability to focus may suffer.

Fortunately, a melatonin supplement may get you back on track. That's according to a study of 104 adults with delayed sleep-wake phase disorder, a condition that causes folks to have trouble going to sleep or getting up on time.

Researchers gave volunteers 0.5 milligram of fast-release melatonin an hour before bedtime for 28 days. The scientists discovered that participants who took the supplement at least five nights in a row each week fell asleep 34 minutes earlier than those taking a placebo. They also slept better and reported improvements in their ability to function at work, school, and at home.

Curious but not ready for a supplement? Try a bedtime snack of melatonin-rich pistachio nuts, milk, oats, or eggs.

Sleeping like a baby helps weight loss. Ever wonder why the popular television show "The Biggest Loser" champions the importance of a good night's rest? It's because obesity has been linked to poor sleep quality. Studies show that a groggy brain tends to crave energy-dense, high-carbohydrate foods. And too little sleep can slow your metabolism, causing you to pack on the pounds.

So if you want better control of your weight, get a handle on your sleep. Melatonin can help with that, according to a monthlong study of 30 people who were obese. Half of them took 10 mg of melatonin an hour before bedtime and followed a calorie-restricted diet. The rest took a placebo while on the same diet. Women ate 1,000 to 1,200 calories a day, while men took in 1,400 to 1,600 calories a day.

Restricting calories helped both groups, but the melatonin group saw greater reductions in body weight and body mass index. The researchers say that may be due to increased levels of adiponectin — a hormone that regulates the metabolism of lipids and glucose — in the volunteers who took melatonin.

If you're ready to eat better for sleep, consider some fish and gluten-free black rice for supper. Or add more melatonin with sides like barley, peppers, tomatoes, and mushrooms.

BRIGHT IDEA

Supplement your snooze with melatonin

You may not realize it, but you probably change your sleep position as many as 60 or 70 times a night. With that much flip-flopping, no wonder some folks wake up unexpectedly. Sleep experts offer plenty of advice for falling and staying asleep — everything from playing soothing sounds to buying a new mattress. But if you've tried such self-help tips with no success, it may be time to get the lowdown on melatonin supplements.

While short-term melatonin use is generally considered safe for healthy adults, you should only take it as needed. Start with the lowest dose of 1 milligram (mg) or less about 45 minutes before bedtime. If that's not quite enough, try 3 mg. Taking more than that — 5 mg or 10 mg, for example — may be more than you need.

It's important to proceed with caution when buying melatonin. A study published in the *Journal of Clinical Sleep Medicine* found that the melatonin content of supplements varied widely. More than 70% of tested products failed to meet a 10% margin of the amount declared on the label. The actual melatonin content ranged from 83% less to 478% more than claimed.

That's why you should look for the "USP Verified" mark, which indicates that the supplement meets formula requirements set by the U.S. Pharmacopeial Convention.

Memory tools

6 techniques to sharpen your recall

"Memory is the treasury and guardian of all things." This quote is attributed to the famous Roman scholar and orator Cicero. Although your memory won't last over 2,000 years, like Cicero's preserved speeches, you can train it to remember information more easily with these six techniques.

Piggyback. Help your recall by linking fresh material to an already established memory. Want to remember your neighbor is from New York? Think about your trip to the Big Apple and connect the two.

Rehearse, recall, repeat. Ever forget someone's name right after you met them? How embarrassing! You're not alone, though. People may forget as much as 80% of newly learned information within a few days. But repetition can help you retrieve the information later on.

So next time you meet someone, say their name out loud and repeat it several times in the conversation. Or try subbing them into "The Name Game," song from the 1960s. "Shirley, Shirley, bo-ber-ley, bo-na-na fanna, fo-fer-ley, fee fi mo-mer-ley, Shirley!" Who could forget a name after that?

Memory palace. Be like Sherlock Holmes and use this strategy also called the method of loci — to make your memories stick.

Start by picking a familiar place, like your house or a well-known street, to be your "palace." Then map a route through the space, placing the information you want to remember in distinct spots as you walk through. You'll follow this path each time to keep those memory triggers in order.

Maybe you want to remember your sister lives in Chicago. Using a mind palace of your childhood home, you could envision the city's famous sculpture, "The Bean," sitting on an armchair. When you imagine walking through your palace, you'll see the silver sculpture and remember Chicago.

Chunking. Birds of a feather flock together. And the same is true of information if you want to remember it more easily. Instead of memorizing individual items, group related things together under a new name. Milk, butter, and yogurt on your shopping list become "dairy."

It works for numbers, too. For instance, 46718035 becomes 46-71-80-35. Experts often recommend using three to seven chunks.

Mind mapping. Students draw these idea organizers to help them learn material, but you can use them in your daily life, too. Begin with a central idea in the middle and branch related information from that main concept to create subtopics. Link branches together to connect ideas or add subbranches to expand even more.

This method illustrates the connections between ideas you're trying to remember and offers you more flexibility than a list. Later, you can guide your mind through the different connections to help with recall.

Visualize and peg. You won't leave the store without items you need when you use the rhyming peg system to memorize lists. Start by learning the "pegs." Each number, one through 10, is assigned a rhyming word. One pairs with bun, two with shoe, three with tree, and so on. Vividly imagine each rhymed word.

Then take the items on your shopping list and match them to your pegs. If you want to remember orange juice, for example, link it to three/tree by imagining oranges growing on a tree in your grocery store.

Want to take your learning up a notch? Become the teacher for a day. Called the protege effect, researchers have discovered that explaining a topic to someone else improves your understanding and recall. You'll pick out and organize the most important information and find gaps in your own thinking.

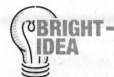

Tracking down lost objects is as easy as 1-2-3

Searching for lost items? There's more to it than meets the eye — literally. When scanning the room for an object, say, your sweater, your brain takes into account its softness and skips past hard things. So even though you may consciously be thinking about its color and size, your brain is automatically sorting traits you don't see.

Your brain's intuitive search feature isn't always enough, though. This simple three-step process is all you need to find most things right off the bat.

Step 1. Stay calm. You'll find what you've mislaid more efficiently if you take a deep breath and focus.

Step 2. Retrace your steps. Make a vivid mental picture of the last time you saw the object, and you may trigger details that reveal its location. Then double-check in and around the area you last used the rogue item. Objects tend to drift less than 1 1/2 feet from their normal place.

Step 3. Stop searching all over for things you misplace. Lost belongings seem to disappear to the same room — the messiest — so if you're not sure where you last saw your item, search the most cluttered space. Save your room from falling into greater disarray by sorting what you've already looked at from what's left.

Bonus — make things easier to spot. A chunky keychain or bright sticky note make your keys and important papers stand out. And if you reduce clutter, valuable items will have fewer opportunities to get lost in the jumble.

Fantastic 4: Old-school memory tools that really work

Ever feel like your brain sprung a leak and now your whole grocery list has washed away? These classic memory tools put a stopper in your mind. So break out your pencil for some tried-and-true tactics.

Use flash cards. Whether you're waiting in line or riding the subway, you always have time to learn with this portable tool. It uses a process called spaced repetition — meaning you review material at gradually lengthening intervals. With normal study techniques, you may find yourself dumping the information soon after. But practicing information recall over increasing spans of time helps your brain pack it in for the long term.

This tactic began in the '70s with the Leitner system, but you can go digital with a variety of apps and websites. They'll vary how often different material pops up depending on its difficulty.

Handwrite notes. Researchers say writing by hand makes it easier for you to learn and remember new information.

Through the act of writing, touching the paper, and holding the pencil, your brain gets feedback that helps strengthen the memory process. When you type on a keyboard, you don't get the same brain-boosting results.

Draw pictures. A picture is worth a thousand words, so the saying goes. And when it comes to remembering, that seems to hold true. Researchers have found that drawing pictures helps you hold on to twice as much information as writing the words down. That's because your hand's motion as it makes pencil strokes, combined with the visual depiction, help ingrain the idea.

Don't try to take a shortcut, though. Researchers have shown drawing helps your memory more than imagining the object or describing it. You don't have to be an artist to benefit, either. Just take four seconds to doodle an image, and enjoy the results.

Come up with rhymes or acronyms. Make remembering a game with acronyms and rhymes. First write down your grocery list and highlight the first letter of each item. If any words jump out at you, make them your acronym. For instance, carrots, apples, and tea become CAT. If not, group them the best you can into a nonsense word you can remember. Spinach, peaches, eggs, rice, and yogurt become SPERY or RYPSE.

Rhymes can help information stay intact, too. After all, you probably still know the catchy reminder "I before E except after C" from grammar school.

Improve your memory with these 11 effective remedies

You may feel like you've reached your brain's capacity when things start slipping through the cracks. But you really can remember more. The secrets you learned in this chapter can help maximize your memory.

- Piggyback new information onto an established memory.

- Repeat names shortly after an introduction to help with recall.

- Build a memory palace in your mind to store information.

- Group material into chunks and remember those instead of individual details.

- Chart a mind map to make memorable connections between ideas.

- Apply the rhyming peg system to lists for easier memorization.

- Use flash cards to review new information.

- Handwrite notes to strengthen your memory.

- Draw a picture of what you're trying to remember.

- Make up an acronym or rhyming phrase to trigger details.

- Share what you're learning.

MIND diet

Double down on protection with one delightful diet

The old saying is true — you are what you eat. And that's where the MIND — an acronym for the Mediterranean-DASH Intervention for Neurodegenerative Delay — diet comes in. Developed by researchers specifically to improve your brain health, it's a combination of two of the healthiest eating plans.

Much like the Mediterranean and DASH food programs, the MIND diet asks people to eat whole grains and plant-based meals instead of red meat, unhealthy fats, and sugar. However, the MIND diet places a bigger emphasis on foods that ramp up your brainpower, like leafy greens and berries.

Worried about dementia? The MIND diet cuts your risk. If you're not great at restricting what you eat, the MIND diet could be just what you need. Research suggests that you need to commit wholeheartedly to the DASH or Mediterranean diet if you want to get all of the promised brain benefits. But the MIND diet can protect you from Alzheimer's disease (AD) even if you take a few cheat days.

In a study published in the journal *Alzheimer's & Dementia*, researchers pitted the MIND diet against the two meal plans that it's based on. They recruited 923 healthy seniors who were already following the principles of the MIND, Mediterranean, and DASH diets.

The researchers followed the participants over more than four years, noting which ones developed AD. The scientists found that the seniors who strictly stuck to the MIND diet cut their risk of developing AD by as much as 53%. People who closely followed the DASH and Mediterranean diets lowered their risk, too.

However, seniors who weren't as good about following the MIND diet still lowered their risk of AD — by as much as 35%. The same wasn't true for the other two diets. Experts say that could be because the MIND diet puts more emphasis on leafy greens and berries. Studies suggest the nutrients in these foods — including folate, vitamin E, carotenoids, and flavonoids — help protect your brain from dementia.

Ward off cognitive decline with fabulous fare. Feel like old age is catching up with you? The MIND diet could be exactly what you need. A few simple tweaks to your meals could keep your brain fit as a fiddle.

American researchers followed 960 seniors on the MIND diet and found that the volunteers who adhered to the meal plan the most had significantly slower rates of cognitive decline than those who followed it the least. In fact, researchers say the seniors who stuck to the diet appeared to be 7 1/2 years younger cognitively than the other group.

Use your MIND to beat the blues. Here's another reason to try the MIND diet. Research suggests it can help lift your spirits.

In a recently published study, 709 seniors with symptoms of depression logged the details of their diets. Researchers then tracked their moods over more than six years. The scientists found that the people who strongly complied with the MIND diet had lower rates of depressive symptoms than those who followed it the least. In contrast, people who ate a Western-style diet — one that's rich in unhealthy fats, red meat, and prepackaged foods — had higher rates of depression.

Researchers think that fiber from the vegetables and whole grains in this diet may help fight inflammation, which has been linked to depression.

Shopping for fish? Don't grab any old package. Pollutants, toxins, and other harmful chemicals can build up in large, older fish like swordfish, shark, and king mackerel. Fortunately, you can avoid much of the danger by choosing small fish low in the food chain, like sardines and anchovies. Salmon and pollock are also good choices.

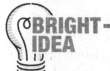

MIND the difference — how do these 3 diets stack up?

The Mediterranean diet, the DASH diet, and the MIND diet all shy away from red meat, sweets, and fatty foods. They also ask you to pile your plate with whole grains, veggies, and other healthy foods. Still, you'll want to know the key differences between the three plans. Here's what you need to know.

	MIND diet	Mediterranean diet	DASH diet
vegetables	at least 1 serving a day	4-8 servings a day	4-5 servings a day
leafy greens	1 serving a day	included with other vegetables	included with other vegetables
fruit	n/a	2-4 servings a day	4-5 servings a day
berries	at least 2 servings a week	included with other fruit	included with other fruit
whole grains	3 or more servings a day	4-6 servings a day	7-8 servings a day
fatty fish	at least 1 serving a week	2-3 servings a week	1-2 servings a day
poultry and lean meat	at least 2 servings a week	1-3 servings a week	1-2 servings a day
beans and other legumes	4 or more servings a week	2-4 servings a day	4-5 servings a week
nuts	at least 5 servings a week	2-4 servings a day	4-5 servings a week
healthy fats	use olive oil	4-6 servings a day	2-3 servings a day

Mint

A tasty way to keep your brain in mint condition

Every year they come to town. Samoas, Tagalongs, shortbread Trefoils. Those tempting, delicious Girl Scout cookies. An estimated 200 million boxes of the tasty treats are sold each year. It probably comes as no surprise that Thin Mints are the most popular, racking up around 25% of total cookie sales. But what makes them such a hit? Maybe the hint of all-natural peppermint oil from the popular herb that is not only delicious, but is brain healthy, too.

Now no one is suggesting you chow down on a dozen boxes of Thin Mints to help you remember your grocery list. But keeping your brain healthy for the long term can be as simple as going to the garden, or your fresh produce aisle, and choosing this one incredible plant — mint.

Tea up for a better memory. Dr. Mark Moss and his associates at Northumbria University conducted a study designed to determine the effects of peppermint tea, chamomile tea, and plain hot water on the mood and memory of 180 people.

The researchers tested the participants' cognition and mood before and after drinking. And they concluded that the peppermint tea improved long-term memory and working memory — which includes skills like reasoning, comprehension, and certain types of learning — compared to chamomile or hot water. Peppermint also increased alertness. Chamomile tea actually slowed memory and produced a calming effect.

"It's interesting to see the contrasting effects on mood and cognition of the two different herbal teas," said Dr. Moss. "The enhancing and arousing effects of peppermint and the calming, sedative effects of chamomile observed in this study are in keeping with the claimed properties of these herbs and suggest beneficial effects can be drawn from their use."

Improving recall is all in the family. The plant family *Lamiaceae*, that is. Researchers aren't really sure why peppermint helps with memory. But in one study, they found that spearmint extract, a close cousin to peppermint, did improve working memory in seniors with age-related memory problems. They point to studies that say these brain benefits might come from the polyphenols that are found in plants belonging to the *Lamiaceae* family, like peppermint and spearmint.

Freshly minted cures come from this sweet leafy green

According to Greek myth, the nymph Minthe nearly met her death when angry goddess Persephone discovered the nymph's crush on her hubby, Hades. In fact, Persephone was about to pound her rival into the ground — literally — when Hades turned Minthe into a mint plant to protect her. Not much of a hero.

But since that ancient argument, mint has become a symbol of hospitality and wisdom. It has also received accolades as an herb with a wellspring of healing powers.

Sweet dreams are made of this. Studies show that a lack of sleep increases your risk of high blood pressure, heart disease, and diabetes. And experts know sleep deprivation

Have you ever been in charge of the children's choir on Christmas Eve? Certainly a challenging task. Legend says that in 1670, a desperate German choirmaster gave white candy sticks shaped like shepherds' crooks to his wiggly singers, hoping to calm them. The traditional peppermint flavor and red stripes weren't added until the 20th century.

hinders learning, slows your reaction time, and impairs your cognitive performance.

So researchers studied the effects of spearmint extract on men and women, 50 to 70 years old, with age-related cognitive decline. Each day over the three-month test period, seniors received either 900 or 600 milligrams (mg) of spearmint extract or a placebo. Compared to those who took a placebo, those who took the 900 mg reported they found it easier to get to sleep.

The minty cure that can calm irritable bowel syndrome (IBS). If you're among the estimated 10% to 15% of people affected by IBS worldwide, you may already know the diarrhea, constipation, fatigue, and difficulty sleeping brought on by this condition. And oddly enough, it's not just your gut that's in trouble.

Your brain and your gut are intimately connected. Ever felt butterflies in your stomach? Your head lets the intestines know there's a problem, and your intestines do the same for the brain. Your stomach can signal your mind to feel anxiety, stress, or depression. But studies also show peppermint oil can calm your troubled tummy.

In a study in the Netherlands, researchers found that the kind of peppermint oil capsules that break down in the small intestines reduced the severity of IBS symptoms. Be sure to choose this type — called enteric-coated capsules — when you purchase peppermint oil in pill form. The coating prevents your stomach acids from releasing the oil into your stomach. And that can prevent side effects like heartburn, nausea, and worsening reflux symptoms.

Stem headache pain with this natural healer. Treating tension headaches with peppermint oil has proven to be more effective than placebos in controlled studies.

Peppermint oil is called a "hot" oil, which means you'll feel a warm sensation when you apply it to your skin. Start out by using the oil mixed in a 1-to-4 ratio with a carrier oil such as jojoba or almond oil. Or if you prefer to use it undiluted, use one drop on your skin just to see how it feels. If you have a reaction to the oil, dilute it and try again.

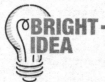

BRIGHT IDEA

More than just juleps: Fancy up your menu with mint

Did you know the Kentucky Derby was started in 1875 by Meriwether Lewis Clark, William Clark's grandson — yes, that William Clark of the Lewis and Clark expedition? Traditions abound around this race, like wearing elaborate hats or drinking the race's official beverage, the Mint Julep.

Legend says Clark grew fresh mint for his juleps just outside the racetrack's clubhouse, but Mint Juleps didn't become the official Derby cocktail until 1939. Try using this versatile herb to create your own delicious traditions.

Caring for mint is a cinch. Mint plants are easy to care for, but raise them in pots rather than in the ground because mint can easily take over your garden. Mint grows best in light soil with good drainage and full sun to partial shade.

Buying at the supermarket instead? Choose leaves that are bright and blemish-free. Store the leaves in a plastic bag in the fridge for up to one week. Or combine chopped mint with water in an ice cube tray and freeze.

Mix up some minty memories. Try these unforgettable mint treats your family will love.

- Whip up a mint limeade by combining lime juice, sugar, and mashed mint leaves.

- Freshen up plain water by adding a little mint and cucumber.

- Lift the flavor of salads, Greek yogurt, or fresh pineapple with chopped mint.

- For a delicious tea, pour hot water over mint leaves and steep for five to six minutes.

- Try new varieties — chocolate mint, orange mint, ginger mint, apple mint, and more. The flavors reflect their namesakes.

Mushrooms

Make mushrooms a mealtime priority for your mind

Fungi eat rocks. That's right. They release natural acids that dissolve rock and mine it for nutrients like potassium, calcium, and magnesium. Certain fungi even pass those nutrients along to people through their fruit — mushrooms.

And edible mushrooms might get pretty close to being a perfect superfood. They pack in lots of good stuff your body needs, like B vitamins, potassium, and fiber. Plus they're fat free, gluten free, cholesterol free, low in calories, and low in sodium. And there's a bonus. They may help you flex your mental muscles.

Shifts or problems with memory, language, attention, and visual-spatial thinking can be early warning signs of mild cognitive impairment (MCI). These changes may not disrupt everyday activities, but they are noticeable.

But mushrooms might lower your risk of MCI, according to researchers in Singapore. How? Helpful compounds in mushrooms may limit the creation of proteins that cause damaging plaques and tangles to form in the brain over time.

The scientists surveyed how often 663 seniors ate mushrooms as part of their regular diet. Some of the participants had MCI while the majority had normal mental function. After six years, researchers found that seniors who ate 3/4 cup of mushrooms more than twice a week had lower odds of developing MCI. In fact, they were half as likely to have the condition compared to those who ate mushrooms less than once per week.

Could 'shrooms dampen diabetes symptoms?

Fireflies and certain mushrooms have an illuminating trait in common. About 80 varieties of mushrooms give off beautiful glow-in-the-dark hues thanks to a chemical reaction. The critical compounds involved? The molecule luciferin and its enzyme partner, luciferase.

Scientists have used this reaction in animal studies to light up tissues, helping them better understand human diseases. But your health doesn't have to wait for researchers to perfect the technology. You can eat more of the regular varieties of mushrooms to give yourself an advantage over conditions like diabetes.

That's good news because high blood sugar can injure the inside of your artery walls, leading to plaque deposits and reduced blood flow. Impaired blood flow increases your risk of a stroke or heart attack. But mushrooms may help in two ways.

- An early study shows that white button mushrooms could reduce risk factors like inflammation and oxidative stress that contribute to diabetes. People with metabolic syndrome — a collection of symptoms that can lead to diabetes and heart disease — ate mushrooms for 16 weeks. After, their blood samples revealed that levels of an amino acid from mushrooms called ergothioneine, which acts as an antioxidant, doubled. Researchers found other positive changes that suggested anti-inflammatory and antioxidant activity, too.

- Soon people with diabetes may crave oyster mushrooms for more than their savory flavor. Researchers in a clinical trial tested freeze-dried oyster mushroom powders in people with and without diabetes. Both experienced a drop in blood sugar levels after meals, and people with diabetes saw improvements in their insulin levels.

> Dried mushrooms make great kitchen staples. They hold their rich, savory flavor over their long shelf life of two to three years. Soak them in water until they're tender before cooking them. When you strain out the mushrooms, don't forget to use the flavorful broth, too. It's tasty in soups, stews, and sauces.

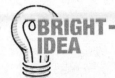

Preserve and prepare your mushrooms like a pro

Get your chicken cliches ready, because you'll need them to describe the *Laetiporus* category of edible mushrooms. Some common names include "chicken of the woods" and "chicken mushroom." And if you're curious to try them, expect these 'shrooms to "taste like chicken."

Mushroom monikers and overused sayings can be fun, but what's really important is that your mushrooms don't taste as tired as cliches sound. So get ready to add a feather to your cap for learning the secret to storing, cleaning, and cooking tasty mushrooms.

Fresh mushrooms come packed with moisture. In fact, that's 85% to 95% of their content. Here's how to keep the moisture balanced until you're ready to eat them.

- Store packaged mushrooms in their original containers and wrappings. Drop loose mushrooms in a brown paper bag. They usually stay fresh on a shelf in your fridge — not the crisper — for about a week.

- Your mushrooms cave under peer pressure. Separate them from strong-smelling foods like garlic and onions so they won't absorb the odors.

- Getting hungry for those mushrooms? Give them a quick rinse with cool water. Pat them dry before cooking.

- Your mushrooms will give off a lot of moisture as they cook. Don't crowd them too tightly with other foods so they can cook down.

- You can do just about anything with fresh mushrooms. Add some variety to your menu by trying them cooked in different ways — stuffed, creamed, roasted, boiled, baked, or fried.

Music therapy

Turn it up! Hear how your favorite tunes keep your brain sharp

Have you heard that music offers a multitude of health benefits? In fact, doctors are prescribing music as a natural remedy for the treatment of Alzheimer's, Parkinson's, depression, and stroke.

Music therapy goes beyond casual listening. It's the clinical use of music — including singing and playing instruments — to restore physical, emotional, and cognitive health. Here's what music therapy can do for you.

Hit the right notes against Alzheimer's disease (AD). You don't need to be a maestro to push back against dementia. A study published in the *Journal of Alzheimer's Disease* suggests a little karaoke will do. Researchers split 298 seniors with AD into three groups and tested their cognitive abilities. Over 90 days, the participants spent an hour a day either singing songs in music therapy sessions, reading the lyrics to songs, or not receiving either new treatment.

When tested again, the singers with mild AD performed better on memory and language tests than the other groups. This may be because singing combines melody and lyrics, two types of information that are stored separately. This may boost your ability to retrieve memories.

Rhythm helps beat back Parkinson's symptoms. Parkinson's disease (PD) is a progressive disorder that affects nerve cells deep in the brain. Symptoms include tremors, slowed movements, and loss of balance.

Luckily, rhythmic auditory exercises — a technique that provides cues like a repeated musical beat to prompt the use of motor skills —

have been shown to improve the symptoms of PD. Many studies suggest such treatment can improve the gait, coordination between limbs, posture, and balance of people with this condition.

Tune in to a better mood and memory. The power of music struck a chord with Hippocrates, the father of Greek medicine who played music to help treat his patients. That interest in music as medicine hasn't faded with falling empires.

In one study, a small group of older adults who reported experiencing cognitive decline sat with their eyes closed for 12 minutes daily as they listened to masterpieces by composers like Bach and Beethoven. After three months, researchers saw marked improvements in their mood and memory. Experts say music ups your brain's production of dopamine, the feel-good chemical that helps regulate your memory and mood.

Scale back stroke damage with music. A stroke can cut off blood circulation and cause brain cells to die. It can be fatal, and survivors can face long-term disability afterward.

But a review of 10 studies of more than 350 people who had suffered a stroke found that music therapy benefits motor skills and executive function, the mental skills you need to manage daily life. Researchers think that music helps with the brain's ability to change and adapt by reorganizing its neurons after injury.

> People with dementia may remember familiar songs well enough to sing along. You can help bring them joy by making a playlist of personalized hits. Top pop songs from their childhood and young adulthood, hymns, and classic singalongs are good choices that may strike a chord with their memories.

Music strikes a high note against pain and insomnia

"I feel good!" James Brown shouts in his 1965 hit "I Got You (I Feel Good)." You'll have no problem matching his enthusiasm, either, when you learn that music can ease your chronic pain and boost your body's ability to ward off insomnia.

Let the music play, chronic pain will drift away. Ever lose track of time listening to a record? That same power that makes time fly can also help dial down your chronic pain. Music changes your perception of pain by taking your focus off your discomfort to make it more manageable.

That benefits your brain, too, because chronic pain may lead to brain activity changes that are connected to depression, anxiety, and difficulty making decisions. Simply listening to music every day can help.

Research suggests musical interventions like passively listening to recorded music provided by a doctor or nurse, as well as the more active music therapy, can ease pain and beat the blues. A review including data from over 3,500 people with cancer found that both uses of music drastically improved the participants' pain levels and even relieved their symptoms of depression.

Participants who experienced both forms of interventions over-whelmingly preferred the music therapy sessions, citing the personal attention and care, the creativity of playing music, and the opportunity to express themselves emotionally.

Float off to sleep on these sound waves. Not getting enough sleep can lead to mood changes and anxiety, which in turn can contribute to problems with memory. But you may be able to avoid all of that by adding some calm songs to your sleep regime. It's enjoyable, and it won't cost a penny.

Forty-five minutes of soothing music before bed is all you need, according to one study. Seniors with insomnia reached deep sleep more quickly, maintained memory-amplifying REM sleep longer, and felt more rested after four nights of this routine than those who didn't listen to music before bed.

Don't worry if you don't have a professional choosing your music. The participants who chose their own bedtime soundtrack experienced the same sleep quality as those who listened to researcher-selected tunes. So if you find it hard to snooze, listen to some blues — or your favorite soothing music — to improve your beauty sleep.

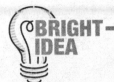

Get rock-star treatment for rock-bottom prices

Remember the petite, bold-voiced singer Teresa Brewer? She belted out "Put another nickel in. In the nickelodeon," way back in 1950. Her top-selling homage to the power of the jukebox was all about playing more "Music! Music! Music!" Fortunately, though, when it comes to music therapy, you don't necessarily have to pay to play.

Medicare. This federal program covers music therapy under its partial hospitalization plan. However, your treatment must meet the following requirements.

- It has to be prescribed by a physician.

- It is reasonable and necessary for your illness or injury.

- It must be goal-oriented and based on a documented treatment plan.

- It will improve — not simply maintain — your current level of functioning.

Medicaid. Funding varies by state. In Texas, for example, music therapy is covered under various Medicaid waiver programs. Even if your state doesn't specifically list music therapy, it may be covered under existing-treatment categories like community support or rehabilitation services.

Private insurance. Providers pay for music therapy on a case-by-case basis. If your program is necessary to reach your treatment goals, your therapy may be covered. Just make sure you have preapproval.

None of these fit your situation? You may also find assistance through your state. Check with your state's departments of mental health or developmental disabilities to start.

Napping

Hit the hay to maximize your memory

A NASA study on pilots found that a 40-minute nap was enough to improve performance by 34%. And what's good for NASA is good for you. Even better? A quick snooze may be exactly what you need to improve your memory.

Take regular naps to rev up your recall. Feeling forgetful? You might just need to sleep it off. A new study published in the *International Journal of Geriatric Psychiatry* revealed that healthy seniors who took regular naps had better memories.

Researchers recruited 2,549 volunteers and asked them if they napped, how often they napped, and how long those naps lasted. The participants also had to clarify whether they planned their naps or nodded off accidentally.

Afterward, researchers put the seniors through a barrage of tests. And they found that those who took 31- to 60-minute naps scored better on memory tests than those who never or rarely took naps. Unintentional naps didn't have the same memory-boosting effects, though. Experts think drifting off to sleep by accident may be a marker of, or a contributor to, poorer cognition among older adults.

Want to remember what you read? Take a power snooze.
Recovery is an essential part of your workout routine. If you don't rest and relax your body while it's tired, you won't get the full benefits from all that exercise. And your brain isn't all that different. Soaking up info is like exercise for your brain. After all that hard work, you need to give it a break.

That's according to a German study of 41 adults who were asked to memorize 90 single words and 120 unrelated word pairs — like "milk-taxi" — that they had never heard together. After being tested on their ability to remember what they had learned, around half of the volunteers took a nap and the rest watched a DVD. The researchers then tested the participants' memories again.

Surprisingly, the people who took naps were able to remember significantly more word pairs compared with the DVD watchers. Researchers say the nappers' performance after sleeping was just as good as it had been right after they first studied the words.

Experts think your brain needs sleep to sort your memories into long-term storage. Scans of sleeping people show bursts of activity in the region of the brain responsible for processing and organizing memories, the researchers say.

Perk up your post-doze mind with this simple trick

Coffee and naps seem like they'd go together about as well as oil and water. After all, most people load up on caffeine so they don't get drowsy. But experts say this dynamic duo is a perfect way to amp up your energy.

The trick is to drink coffee before you settle down for a short snooze. After you finish your cup of joe, set an alarm to wake you up in 20 minutes. The reason? It takes that amount of time for your brain to absorb caffeine.

Here's the scoop. You get tired when a chemical compound called adenosine builds up in your brain. Sleeping clears the adenosine away, making room for caffeine to stimulate your brain when it gets there.

The end result? You get the best of both worlds — a refreshing catnap followed by a caffeinated burst of energy.

High blood pressure? Treat it with an afternoon snooze

High blood pressure can damage your brain in a few ways. It's a major risk factor for stroke, which is sometimes called a "brain attack." When you have a stroke, blood vessels either burst or become blocked. This causes brain cells to die. What's more, several studies have linked high blood pressure to mental decline and memory problems.

Fortunately, though, grabbing forty winks could help keep your blood pressure under control.

In a new study, researchers recruited 212 people with an average age of 62. They split the participants into two groups — one that practiced midday napping and the other that didn't.

The scientists measured the participants' blood pressure, cardiovascular health, physical activity, and how long they napped over a 24-hour period. They found that those who napped had an average systolic blood pressure that was 5.3 mmHg lower than those who didn't. That's about what you could expect from making lifestyle changes or taking blood pressure medication, the scientists say.

Of course, the research results don't mean you should toss out your prescriptions. But it does give you a good excuse to take an afternoon snooze. Experts say the seniors in this study napped for 49 minutes, on average.

"These findings are important because a drop in blood pressure as small as 2 mmHg can reduce the risk of cardiovascular events such as heart attack by up to 10%," says Dr. Manolis Kallistratos, cardiologist at the Asklepieion General Hospital in Voula, Greece, and one of the study's co-authors. "Based on our findings, if someone has the luxury to take a nap during the day, it may also have benefits for high blood pressure. Napping can be easily adopted and typically doesn't cost anything."

> Midday naps are a time-honored tradition. The Spanish word "siesta" actually stems from the Latin term *hora sexta*. This phrase, which literally means sixth hour, refers to the hottest part of the day. That's when farmers traditionally took a post-lunch snooze before returning to work.

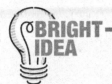

Rude awakening — top tips for outsmarting nap traps

An afternoon nap is more than a way to relax and recharge on a sleepy Sunday. But if you want all the benefits of a midday snooze, you'll need to make sure you're paying attention to a few basic do's and don'ts.

- Don't oversleep. Dozing too long can be a surefire way to ruin your nap. You'll wake up groggy, plus you're almost guaranteed to have a bad night's rest. Try to keep your naps under an hour. Set an alarm so you don't oversleep, or ask a family member to wake you at a certain time.

- Sleep upright if you don't want to fall into a deep sleep. Why not try nestling into your favorite armchair if you're a heavy sleeper? Experts say lying down makes it easier to drift into deep sleep, so snoozing in a chair can help you take shorter naps.

- Time your naps right. Napping too close to bedtime can wreak havoc on your sleep schedule. But how do you know when to take a siesta? Experts say the best time to catch some ZZZs depends on when you start your day. If you get up early, take a snooze around 1 p.m. Late risers should aim for 3 p.m.

- Dreaming during your nap? That's a sign you're not getting enough sleep at night. A nap shouldn't give your body enough time to slip into REM sleep, which is when most dreams occur.

- You shouldn't doze off during the day if you suffer from sleep disorders like insomnia or sleep apnea. Naps can make these conditions worse.

Niacin

B3 — a boon for your brain and body

Ever heard of a pellagrin? No, not the large water bird, pelican. A pellagrin is actually a person who has pellagra, a disease with symptoms like dermatitis, diarrhea, and dementia caused by low levels of vitamin B3. Is this vitamin, also called niacin, not on your radar? It should be.

Like the other B vitamins, vitamin B3 helps your body change carbohydrates into sugar for fuel. That means it plays a big role in cranking up your energy. Think of vitamin B3 like a car's engine. The food you eat is the gas that makes the car (your body) run. But you need something to help convert that gas into mechanical power. Niacin sets off the chemical reactions that transform food into the energy that keeps you going.

This nutrient is so powerful it also helps fortify your mind, manage your cholesterol, and protect your vision.

A lack of niacin meddles with your mind. Your body makes niacin from the essential amino acid tryptophan. But you also get it from foods like beef, turkey, salmon, and avocados. In addition, many grains are enriched or fortified with niacin.

While you might not worry about being low in this vitamin, it's not a bad idea to take inventory of what you eat to see if you're getting enough. Men over age 50 need 16 milligrams and women over 50 need 14 milligrams of niacin a day.

Your brain will be happy to know that scientists think niacin may protect you from age-related cognitive decline and dreaded diseases like Alzheimer's and Parkinson's. Neurons in your brain use this vitamin for energy to help with important functions such as learning and remembering information.

Can't stand statins? B3 steps up for cholesterol control.

Doctors used to prescribe niacin alongside cholesterol medications called statins. By 2013, niacin sales exceeded $1 billion, but the practice has changed.

In a recent review of 17 clinical trials researchers concluded that niacin may have a role in controlling lipid levels — like cholesterol and triglycerides — but only when you can't take standard cholesterol-lowering medication. Their study covered 17,105 people who received niacin supplements and 18,655 participants who got a placebo or a therapy used for lowering cholesterol.

If you are unable to take a statin, a doctor might consider a prescription-strength niacin supplement as a way to tackle high lipid levels, which is linked to heart disease and Alzheimer's.

Don't lose sight of your need for niacin

Snap. Your camera shutter closes on the perfect sunset. You pull up the picture only to be disappointed. Humidity fogged up your lens. The picture is fuzzy and there's no fix for it.

You could always take another picture, but imagine the frustration of having blurry vision all the time with no way to regain clarity. If your optic nerve — the one that connects your eye to your brain — gets damaged from a disease like glaucoma, then you could be stuck with that situation.

Some people with glaucoma notice a gradual loss of side vision, but others see glares or need additional light to see. The condition can cause permanent damage or even blindness. Unfortunately it's also linked to a higher risk of developing Alzheimer's.

Anyone could get glaucoma. But what causes it?

- Pressure changes inside the eye can occur when drainage canals get clogged or blocked. You may not even realize this is happening.

- Family history makes you more susceptible to glaucoma. Since you might not have any symptoms at all, it is important to get regular eye exams.

- Poor nutrition — like being low in niacin — is also associated with glaucoma.

Luckily, boosting B3 through your diet is pretty simple. And niacin-rich foods are a feast for your eyes. Here's what the experts say.

See the difference niacin makes. Researchers have recently discovered some eye-opening benefits of vitamin B3. They analyzed nutrients from the diets of nearly 17,000 people in Korea to see how niacin might affect the risk of developing glaucoma. During this four-year study, the scientists collected information through food surveys and ranked it by nutrients.

Results showed that participants who ate more niacin-rich foods daily were less likely to develop glaucoma. This held true even when researchers removed the data for people who took niacin supplements.

Step up your B3 quota. You might not be getting enough niacin if you restrict your diet for digestive conditions like Crohn's disease. Or if you follow a strict gluten-free, vegetarian, or vegan diet, you have to be intentional about eating foods with niacin.

What can you eat to boost your niacin? Half a roasted chicken breast meets 74% of the daily niacin needs for a man age 50 or above. But a can of tuna nets even more at 113%.

If you prefer plants, keep those legumes coming. Asian food features niacin in tempeh — a soy product — and peanut dishes. You could also serve up portobello mushrooms or snack on pumpkin seeds.

Next time you're shopping the meat aisle, do a quick comparison of the labels for the plant-based meat substitute Impossible Burger and regular ground beef. You might be surprised to see the nutritional differences. The Impossible Burger touts nearly as much protein as well as more minerals, fiber, and vitamins like niacin.

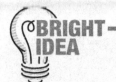

Fortified cereals get you far-out nutrition

Even after Neil Armstrong, Buzz Aldrin, and Michael Collins took those first steps on the moon in 1969, they still needed some breakfast. Zero gravity wasn't friendly to milk, but they had little space-age cereal cubes.

Back then you could even play astronaut games on the backs of your cereal boxes while you ate your breakfast. And the same cereal the moonwalkers got helped you start your day with vitamins like niacin. You still need those nutrients today.

Fortified cereals make an affordable, easy solution for getting vitamins into your diet — including niacin. But it can be hard to find the right balance between flavor and nutrition. Tasty varieties may have 100% of some of the vitamins you need daily, but they may also have an unhealthy amount of sugar.

Thankfully it's not rocket science to figure out which ingredients need to show up in your breakfast food. Look for whole grains, fiber, and low or no sugar on the label.

You might be wondering which cereals meet your niacin needs and still keep the sugar in check. Here are some top contenders, along with the percent of the daily recommended amount of niacin a serving offers women over 50.

- Ralston Enriched Bran Flakes — 188%

- General Mills Whole Grain Total — 143%

- Kellogg's All-Bran Complete Wheat Flakes — 143%

- Ralston Tasteeos — 51%

- General Mills Cheerios — 38%

If cereal isn't your thing, you could mix up a tasty pack of low-sugar, fortified instant oatmeal, which still gets you 39% of a woman's daily niacin.

Nuts and seeds

Put the 'nut' in nutrition with these 4 fabulous seeds

"Sometimes you feel like a nut. Sometimes you don't," crooned the Almond Joy folks of long ago. So the almond — seed or nut? It's a seed! Most nuts are seeds, but not all seeds are nuts. Huh? Nuts are the dry fruit of certain plants. They're wrapped in a hard shell. Seeds are immature plants surrounded by seed coats. Both contain protein, vitamins, and minerals.

And one of these seeds even has bragging rights to a magic bullet — an anti-aging nutrient that most people never try. Ready to give it a shot?

This miracle mineral in Brazil nuts makes you feel young again. The mineral is called selenium, and it's abundant in Brazil nuts. Selenium is packed full of antioxidants — the substances that protect your cells from damage. Researchers have long suspected that a low level of antioxidants goes hand in hand with cognitive decline. So they measured the amount of selenium in the blood of 27 seniors with Alzheimer's disease (AD) and 17 with mild cognitive impairment (MCI). A control group of 28 older adults had no cognitive issues.

Nearly everyone in the three groups tested below accepted levels of selenium. The AD group showed the lowest levels, while the MCI group tested slightly higher. Those in the control group had the highest amounts. The researchers concluded that the participants' selenium levels decreased as cognitive function worsened.

They also proposed that a lack of selenium contributes to cognitive decline. The scientists recommended that older folks eat Brazil nuts to restore deficient selenium levels.

Another one of selenium's superpowers? Its potent antioxidants are known to boost your immune system by lowering oxidative stress in your body. Oxidative stress can speed up the aging process and may even contribute to the development of AD and Parkinson's disease.

Sunflower seeds and almonds keep your mind up to speed.
Are you a fan of almonds? How about sunflower seeds? If so, then you're going to love this news. Both seeds are packed full of vitamin E, which may reduce your risk of cognitive decline.

A study of nearly 15,000 women between the ages of 70 and 79 found that those who took vitamin E supplements performed modestly better on cognitive tests than those who never took them. Separate research has found that vitamin E may encourage healthy brain aging and delay the cognitive decline of AD.

PUFAs in walnuts perk up the brain. What are PUFAs? They're polyunsaturated fatty acids. One type of this good fat — omega-3 fatty acids — may slow the development of cognitive diseases. Researchers tested this theory by conducting a two-year study of 636 seniors. Some participants supplemented their diets with 1 to 2 ounces of walnuts — between 14 and 28 walnut halves — per day. The rest didn't.

Study results suggest that the adults who were most at risk at the beginning of the study — those who smoked or had lower neuropsychological test scores — saw cognitive benefits. The researchers say this indicates that walnuts may decrease the risk of cognitive decline in people at higher risk.

> Brazil nuts are bursting with brain-fortifying selenium. So how many should you eat every day — 10, 20, 30? How about one? That's right. Just one Brazil nut provides 68 to 91 micrograms (mcg) of selenium, more than the daily recommended 55 mcg recommended for adults over age 50.

Go nuts to lower your risk of heart disease and diabetes

First the bad news. Nearly 7 out of 10 seniors with diabetes die from some sort of heart disease. A pretty scary stat, wouldn't you say? But don't give up just yet. You can protect yourself.

Now, are you looking for the good news? Here it comes, in a nutshell.

Nuts curb your risk of heart disease. In a decades-long study that included more than 200,000 people, researchers made the simple discovery that folks who ate nuts five or more times every week had a 20% lower risk of coronary heart disease when compared to those who rarely or never ate nuts.

And if your nut of choice is a walnut, you'll be delighted to hear that people who ate more than three 1-ounce servings of this nut each week — that's a total of 21 whole walnuts — had a 47% lower risk of dying from cardiovascular disease (CVD) than those who didn't eat walnuts. Even eating walnuts just once a week lowered the risk of developing CVD by 19%.

Nuts work for you by lowering harmful inflammation, which can lead to heart disease. Inflammation can also raise your risk for developing Alzheimer's disease and other neurodegenerative conditions. So not only are nuts good for your heart, but they help your brain stay healthy, too.

Crack open some diabetes defense. Researchers in India discovered that adding almonds to your diet may be just what you need to control your blood sugar. They studied 50 adults with type 2 diabetes to see how eating whole raw almonds every day for 24 weeks would affect their blood sugar.

At the end of the study, researchers saw that the people who ate almonds had significantly lower HbA1C scores. Those are the numbers that show your average blood sugar level over the past three months. Reductions in HbA1C are important because they indicate a lower risk of developing diabetic complications like heart disease, nerve damage, depression, and Alzheimer's disease.

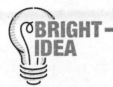

Flax facts: How to bag big benefits from one tiny seed

Flaxseed is truly a wonder food. It protects your brain and heart by lowering blood pressure and cholesterol. And it can reduce your risk of certain types of cancer, too. That's all pretty amazing, but this seed fights arthritis, stomach disorders, and mental problems as well! And women, add just a bit of flaxseed to meals each day to help you deal with menopause symptoms — without the dangerous side effects of hormone replacement therapy.

Discover new ways to use flaxseed, the miracle healer.

Give your meals some flax appeal. Sprinkle ground flaxseed over your breakfast cereal or blend it into your morning smoothie. Mix it into lunchtime soups or stews. Delicious! Or roast whole flaxseeds in a skillet and grind before adding to your dinner salad.

Out of eggs? Flax to the rescue. To replace one egg in your recipe, blend 2 tablespoons of ground flaxseed with 3 tablespoons of cold water. Let the mixture rest for 10 minutes until it has thickened. Perfect for baking yeast breads, cookies, pancakes, or muffins.

Chill your flax to keep it fresh. To get the longest life out of your flaxseed, store it in the refrigerator or freezer. By keeping ground flaxseed in the fridge, you'll extend its shelf life by one or two months past the expiration date. Freeze it and it will stay fresh up to three months after that date. Whole flaxseed can stay fresh in your freezer for up to a year.

Olive oil

Win the war against cognitive decline with this Mediterranean staple

Olive oil has always held a special place in Mediterranean countries. Some ancient Greeks called it "liquid gold," and they used it in almost everything from food to perfume. The famed physician Hippocrates even thought olive oil could heal cuts and scrapes.

Now, this liquid gold is a staple of the Mediterranean diet, an eating plan that's known to slow brain changes associated with the early development of dementia. But is there something more to this healthy fat? Recently, researchers designed a test to see if olive oil could offer more brain benefits than the Mediterranean diet alone.

In the study, scientists asked 110 seniors to follow the Mediterranean diet for a year. However, half of the people were asked to swap out all the vegetable oils they used for olive oil.

Researchers tested people's cognitive abilities before and after the trial and found that those who ate olive oil every day showed more improvement. The authors think the nutrients in olive oil helped fight inflammation and oxidative stress in the brain that can cause cognitive decline.

Want to try this at home? People in the study ate about 1 1/2 to 2 1/4 tablespoons of olive oil a day. And they used extra-virgin olive oil, which contains more nutrients than light, or refined, olive oil.

While swapping out bad fats for olive oil can take your brainpower to the next level, be careful not to overdo it. All fats are high in calories. You need to get some in your diet, but too much can lead to weight gain.

Want to tackle this triple threat? Opt for olive oil

Simply swapping out a pat of butter for a drizzle of olive oil doesn't seem like it could make a big difference. After all, both of these foods are added fats. But this tiny change can have a tremendous impact on your health. Experts think olive oil may be one of the healthiest fats you can put in your body.

Ticker trouble? Ditch bad fats for a healthier choice. You probably know a diet high in saturated fats — like butter or lard — can put you on the fast track for heart disease. But did you know researchers think people who have a higher risk of heart disease are more likely to experience cognitive decline? There's good news, though. Trading those bad fats for olive oil can slash your risk of heart disease.

A recent, large-scale study published in the *Journal of the American College of Cardiology* reviewed the diets of more than 90,000 men and women for 24 years. And the researchers found that people who ate the most olive oil — at least half a tablespoon a day — had a 14% lower risk of any kind of cardiovascular disease.

Plus replacing a teaspoon of butter, margarine, mayonnaise, or dairy fat with the same amount of olive oil lowered their risk of coronary heart disease — the kind usually caused by plaque buildup in the arteries — by 7%.

"Using vegetable oils in cooking and in salads makes good sense," says Penny Kris-Etherton, Ph.D., R.D.N., professor of nutrition at Pennsylvania State University and chair of the American Heart Association's Lifestyle and Cardio-metabolic Health Council.

"Research has overwhelmingly found that diets that are rich in plant-based foods, including healthier vegetable oils such as olive, safflower, corn, and many others, can significantly benefit heart health," says Kris-Etherton. "Butter and tropical oils (palm oil

> Want to try baking with olive oil instead of butter? A good rule of thumb is to use 3/4 the amount of butter that the recipe calls for. So if a batch of muffins needs 1 cup of butter, you'll only need 3/4 cup of olive oil.

and coconut oil) are both high in saturated fat, which raises LDL cholesterol ('bad cholesterol') in many people. Margarine made with vegetable oil is also a source of healthy fats."

A spoonful of olive oil on the regular can protect your peepers. Researchers have found that taking good care of your eyes may prevent cognitive decline. That's because poor vision may stop you from joining in activities that stimulate your mind. How can you keep your eyesight sharp? Olive oil.

Researchers interviewed 654 seniors to see what types of cooking oil and fats they preferred and how often they used them. And the scientists found that people who regularly used olive oil had a lower risk of late age-related macular degeneration (AMD), which causes blurred or blank spots in your vision.

Experts say olive oil's powers lie with a naturally occurring chemical called oleocanthal, which works a bit like over-the-counter anti-inflammatory drugs. Over time, low doses of oleocanthal may help fight off the chronic inflammation in your body that contributes to diseases like AMD.

Fend off high blood sugar with this surprising food. A diet loaded with fat may not seem like an antidote for high blood sugar, but research says it may be exactly what you need. The trick is choosing a healthy fat, like olive oil.

A small study on adults with prediabetes found that 12 weeks of an olive oil-rich diet improved insulin sensitivity. The more sensitive you are to insulin, the less you have to worry about blood sugar spikes, which can damage your blood vessels and result in poor blood circulation to your brain. That might cause memory loss and difficulty concentrating.

Participants were told to get about 28% of their daily calories from monounsaturated fats — the type of healthy fats found in olive oil, almonds, cashews, pistachios, and avocados. And half of that amount should be olive oil. On a 2,000 calorie a day diet, you'd aim for about 2 1/3 tablespoons of olive oil.

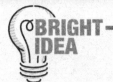

BRIGHT IDEA

3 surefire tips to track down the perfect bottle

Want to wade into the world of olive oil but don't know were to start? Here's what you need to look for.

- Steer clear of the light stuff. Extra-virgin olive oil has the most antioxidants and polyphenols. But light or just plain olive oil has been processed and refined, which strips away most of the health benefits.

- Darker is better. Next time you're choosing an olive oil, pay attention to the color of the bottle. Light causes the nutrients to break down, so it's best to look for dark glass bottles or metal tins. Some clear bottles are OK, provided they're stored in boxes or out of the light before you buy them. But stay away from plastic.

- Check out the harvest date. Does the label have one listed? Eureka. It's likely a higher quality oil. In general, the oil keeps for two years after the harvest date.

- Pay attention to the flavor. Some specialty shops give you the option to taste olive oils before you buy them. But how do you know what you're looking for? The antioxidants and polyphenols give olive oil a peppery, almost bitter, bite. Milder tasting oils won't pack quite the same antioxidant punch. If the flavor is a bit too much for you to handle, try pairing it with strongly flavored dishes like garlicky pasta.

Optimism

Promote brain health with the power of positive thinking

Optimism and pessimism are two different ways of viewing the world. You may recall the common comparison that optimists see the glass half full, a positive outlook, and pessimists see the glass half empty, a focus on the negative. You might not feel just one way all of the time, but you can improve your mindset even if you tend to be more pessimistic. And that brings along a boatload of brain benefits.

Optimism helps you grow old with a better brain. According to researchers, staying positive may be the next great way to maintain mental skill as you age. In a study of over 4,000 couples, scientists found a positive association between personal optimism and both memory and ability to process information.

You're not alone in the fight, though. Having an optimistic partner at your side is healthier for your brain.

The effect of positivity on physical health is threefold. An upbeat attitude may encourage healthy lifestyle choices like eating a balanced diet and regularly exercising.

"We spend a lot of time with our partners," says William Chopik, co-author of the couples study. "They might encourage us to exercise, eat healthier, or remind us to take our medicine. When your partner is optimistic and healthy, it can translate to similar outcomes in your own life. You actually do experience a rosier future by living longer and staving off cognitive illnesses."

It may also affect brain-related processes like autonomic functioning, which involves blood flow and other involuntary activities. And a bright outlook can promote quality social interactions that help you maintain good health.

Look on the bright side of aging to lower your risk of dementia. "Do not resent growing old. Many are denied the privilege," goes an Irish proverb. Easier said than done, perhaps, but research suggests having a positive attitude about aging is good for you and may protect against dementia. Negative thinking, on the other hand, is linked to worse brain function and the buildup of harmful brain proteins linked to Alzheimer's disease.

Researchers found that seniors with a positive perspective about growing older had a 44% lower risk of developing dementia over a four-year study than those with negative beliefs. The results were even stronger among participants who had a gene that increases dementia risk. Those people were 50% less likely to develop dementia than those with negative convictions about aging.

Your mindset may impact your brain because of stress. A negative outlook can increase your stress, which may contribute to the development of dementia.

Update your outlook for internal healing

"It's a beautiful day, don't let it get away." Embracing the good things in life, like the famous Irish rock band U2 advises on their hit "Beautiful Day," is one way you can live a healthier life. Positivity is more than perspective — it's a health tool.

The heart-healing power of hopefulness. "Don't be too hard on yourself," is more than casual advice when it comes to your ticker. Thinking kind thoughts about yourself can calm your heart rate. Plus researchers have found that a cheerful disposition regarding your future is tied to a lower risk of heart disease — a dangerous condition that can damage your blood vessels and disrupt the flow of oxygen-rich blood to your brain.

One group of experts analyzed data on the perspectives of more than 229,000 people. They found that optimism is associated with a lower risk of cardiovascular events, like dying from heart disease, while pessimism is associated with a higher risk. That means upping your optimism may play an important role in preventing life-threatening conditions.

This may be because optimism is linked to healthier diet and exercise habits as well as factors like inflammation and blood vessel function.

Raise your spirits to lower your blood pressure. High blood pressure (HBP) is one of the most common causes of stroke and has long been linked with the development of Alzheimer's disease. But you may be able to protect against the condition by managing your emotions in a healthy way. That's because your feelings can impact your body's response systems — like the sympathetic nervous system — that help control blood pressure.

Experts analyzed how different emotional states impact blood pressure. They found that anxiety and depressive symptoms, like hopelessness or sadness, are associated with a greater risk of HBP. But seeing the world through rose-colored glasses may give your heart a break.

Optimism, a sense of purpose, and emotional vitality, which is an enthusiasm for life, are all components of positive mental well-being. And having those kinds of traits is associated with lower resting blood pressure. Emotional vitality, in particular, has been linked to a lower risk of HBP.

6 ways to grapple with grief

It's difficult to be positive when you're weighed down by grief. But connection and expression can help you buoy your spirits and avoid spiraling into depression. Try these tips to renew your optimism.

- Tell friends and family how you feel. Ask for help if you need it.
- Don't ignore your health. Eat well, exercise, and schedule routine doctor visits. Take your medication.

- Communicate with someone daily. It can be as simple as a phone call or email.

- Find a support group for mourners. Hospitals and religious groups are a good place to start.

- Express your feelings through music, journaling, or painting.

- Seek professional help if you find yourself overwhelmed and unable to perform daily tasks. If left unchecked, grief can lead to depression or worsen the symptoms in someone already depressed.

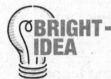

BRIGHT IDEA

How to train your brain to be more optimistic

Fallen into a rut of negative thinking? It may feel inescapable. But changing your perspective is easier than you may expect if you take a little time for self-reflection.

First you have to recognize your negative thoughts. Do you dismiss good things in your life as "lucky" but blame yourself when things go wrong? Challenge that initial pessimistic response by thinking about what outside factors may have had an impact. Examine what underlying beliefs are guiding that response. Then cut off the negative thinking with these activities.

- Keep a journal. Underline the good things that happened during your day and reflect on them.

- Stop negative thoughts short by switching to an enjoyable activity. Listen to music or read a book to shift your attention.

- Maintain your sense of purpose. During retirement you may feel a little lost without a job. Fill your time by trying something new like learning a language or instrument.

- Don't dwell on things out of your control. If global news gets you down, volunteer to help at a local level.

- Be compassionate with yourself. Take time to nurture your body with exercise and a good diet.

- Surround yourself with optimistic people.

Orange juice

Boost your brainpower and slash your risk of stroke

In the early 1970s a South African orange producer called Outspan promoted its fruit throughout Europe with a special orange-shaped car. Only about three still exist, but the message that you should be eating more oranges — and drinking their juice — remains the same. Why? They're good for your mind and body.

Protect your memory with these delicious fruits. Met any flavanones lately? Bet you have. They're compounds found naturally in citrus fruits like oranges and grapefruits. And they have strong antioxidant capabilities that may help prevent damage to brain cells.

Orange juice is loaded with flavanones. And one study at a British university looked at its effects on cognitive function. Researchers recruited 37 healthy seniors and tested their cognitive abilities. Each day for the next eight weeks the volunteers drank either a pint of orange juice mixed with water or a similar-tasting drink low in flavanones. At the end of the study, they found that those who drank the orange juice showed improved performance on cognitive tests compared to those drinking the low-flavanone beverage.

The study suggests that every older American should drink orange juice every day. Experts believe when you do, helpful citrus flavanones called hesperidin and naringenin slide through the protective barrier between your blood and brain. These flavanones may even target learning and memory centers in the brain, the researchers say.

Greatly reduce your stroke risk with orange juice. Older folks fear no condition like stroke, and rightly so. It's a condition that occurs when blood supply to the brain gets blocked or a blood vessel bursts in the brain. And if it happens, immediate medical treatment is vital. But juicy news coming out of a large study in the Netherlands found that a daily 5-ounce glass of orange juice — also rich in vitamin C — can lower stroke risk by nearly one quarter.

Researchers followed nearly 35,000 adults over 15 years, noting how much fruit juice they drank. The scientists compared those figures with the number of strokes that occurred over that period. They discovered that those who drank between four and eight glasses a week of orange or other fruit juices lowered their chances of having a stroke by 24%.

Not a big fan of fruit juice? Those who drank less — between one and four glasses a week — cut their risk by 20%. Just be sure to stick with the no-sugar-added variety.

4 good reasons to snack on oranges

Commercially grown oranges can sit in cold storage for months before finding their way to your grocery store. Even so, you can usually keep them fresh in your refrigerator for up to three weeks. It's good to have a lengthy storage life for a fruit with so many health benefits. So stock up.

An orange a day keeps age-related macular degeneration (AMD) away. Poor vision may prevent you from taking part in activities that stimulate your mind — and that can lead to cognitive decline. AMD is one of the biggest sight stealers among seniors.

But an Australian study of 2,037 older adults found that those who ate at least one orange a day had a 60% lower risk of developing AMD than those who didn't. Folks who ate at least one orange a week also had a reduced risk. The researchers say the flavonoids — phytonutrients with antioxidant powers — in oranges may prevent AMD by warding off cell damage, fighting inflammation, and improving blood flow.

Eat fruit to lower your heart disease risk. As if coronary heart disease isn't bad enough, researchers say it's a risk factor for vascular dementia — a condition that occurs when blood flow to your brain is blocked.

Wouldn't it be great if you could head both diseases off at the pass? Orange juice might help you do just that.

A review of 26 studies found that people who ate between 750 and 800 grams — around 28 ounces — of vitamin C-rich citrus and other fruits a day had a 21% lower risk of developing and dying from heart disease than those who didn't eat any. Sound like a lot of fruit? Eating half that amount cut their chances by more than 15%.

Orange juice squeezes out cholesterol. Too much cholesterol can block your arteries and deprive your brain of the oxygen-rich blood it needs to function.

But a small study found that the juice of blood oranges, which is loaded with a type of flavonoid called anthocyanins, lowered cholesterol levels in women who were obese. Participants drank a cup of juice twice a day over 12 weeks.

Decrease your diabetes risk naturally. Diabetes can damage your blood vessels, putting you at risk for vascular dementia. That's one reason why it's so important to take steps to prevent diabetes.

A study of 24,138 people in China revealed that people who had higher levels of a flavonoid called myricetin in their diet — which they got from foods like oranges — were less likely to develop type 2 diabetes than people with low levels. The researchers say the healthy participants also got their myricetin from apples, peaches, pineapples, and sweet potatoes.

Looking for a hint of orange zest in your drink? After washing and peeling your orange, scrape the bitter white pith away from the rind with a paring knife. Microwave the orange peels for two or three minutes to dry them. Keep the rinds in an airtight jar for easy access, or freeze for later use in sauces, salads, drinks, and more.

Mix it up — try cooking with citrus

Citrus fruits may have cornered the market on versatility in your kitchen. Whatever you're in the mood to make, you can probably pep it up with orange, lemon, lime, or grapefruit — and add a little vitamin C to your dish to boot. Here's how you can put your citrus to work.

- Roast your fruit. Caramelized and mellow citrus sweetness can be yours in just 10 to 15 minutes. Thinly slice the fruit — keep the peel on — and lay it out on parchment paper in a baking pan. Cook the slices at 425 degrees until the edges brown and the juices have leaked out. Roasted orange slices, for example, are a tasty addition to sauteed greens and salads.

- Flavor your food. Meats and vegetables pair well with citrus. Stuff a halved lemon into a whole chicken before roasting. Or cover your baked fish with flavorful grapefruit or lime slices. Feeling adventurous? Use more than one type of citrus.

- Just the juice, ma'am. Even if you don't have a whole orange on hand, you can make clever use of orange juice. Try scrambling an egg with a little OJ for an extra kick. You could also substitute orange juice for water in boxed cake recipes. And OJ ice cubes make your drinks pop. How about a platter of ribs with a citrus tang? Just sprinkle OJ on the meat as it grills. Orange juice also makes a great addition to homemade salad dressing.

Pets

Furry friends fill the bill for better blood pressure and brain function

Pets give you that warm, fuzzy feeling all over. Everyone loves to be welcomed home by a gentle purr, a wagging tail, or a happy horsey nicker. But pets can offer you more than just unconditional love. Through a program called animal-assisted therapy, animals help people cope with heart disease, cancer, mental health disorders, and other health problems.

As Florence Nightingale once said, "A small pet animal is often an excellent companion for the sick."

Going to the dogs lowers your blood pressure. The star of this study was a two-year-old Labradoodle who had been trained to work with residents of nursing homes. The dog's job was to greet each of 15 nursing home residents between the ages of 75 and 100 by placing her head in their laps or by letting them pet her. The seniors also talked to her and played fetch. The visits lasted for 20 minutes.

There were two groups involved in this project — the one that interacted with the therapy dog and researchers and a same-sized control group of nursing home residents that met only with researchers. Both were were divided into even smaller groups, based on the seniors' blood pressure.

Researchers found that the folks with blood pressure greater than or equal to 130 mmHg — considered high blood pressure — saw a significant decrease in heart rate and systolic pressure when they had a dog visit.

That's important because high blood pressure increases your risk of vascular dementia. And the seniors with normal blood pressure and the control group? No change in either blood pressure or heart rate was noted.

How does this work? When the residents were with the dog, researchers think their brain produced oxytocin, one of the "happy hormones" that causes people to enjoy a rush of feel-good emotion.

Oxytocin is known to help lower blood pressure and it's even been compared to an anti-stress medication — without the prescription.

Pets make you happier — and smarter, too. A six-month study of 50 randomly selected folks with Alzheimer's disease (AD) was designed to see how they responded to animal-assisted therapy (AAT).

Participants were divided into three groups. One group received AAT, based on a program called Reality Orientation Therapy (ROT). The program assists people with AD by helping them name objects and people and talk about current and past events. Another group received only ROT treatment, and the control group received neither AAT or ROT.

Both the AAT and ROT folks showed improvements on tests measuring their depression — with the AAT group achieving better results.

The researchers also noted a slight upswing in mood and cognitive function in these two groups. No change was seen in either depression or cognitive function in the control group.

Who can resist a snuggle with a warm puppy? Not 1,500 attendees at an American Heart Association convention in Philadelphia. A fenced play area packed with puppies from a local shelter was set up for folks to enjoy a little cuddle time. The "snuggle zone" was based on research about the heart-healthy connection between people and their pets.

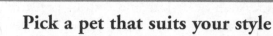

Pick a pet that suits your style

A pet can really spice up a senior's life. Pet owners are more mobile and confident and less lonely. But when it comes to picking a pet, are you barking up the wrong tree? Fido and Fluffy may be just right for some seniors, but there are some downsides, too.

A University of Michigan poll of some 2,000 pet owners between the ages of 50 and 80 found that more than half said pets made it difficult to travel or have fun at events away from home. And some said their pets have caused them to fall or injure themselves.

So before you bring your new pet home, ask yourself some questions.

- What kind of animal fits your home? Will you mind having a little pet hair on the furniture?

- Are you more comfortable adopting an older pet, or would you prefer a younger one?

- What is your activity level? Are you able to move around a lot, or do you spend most of your time resting?

- Do you have the financial resources to care for a pet?

- If you travel, who will take care of your pet?

Consider your pet's needs. All kinds of pets need your attention, like fresh food and water every day. And don't forget those visits to the vet.

- Pick a pup? Dogs require daily outdoor exercise and social interaction. And your dog may benefit from professional training so he understands your expectations.

- Crave a cat? Cats need a clean litter box every day. Daily playtime is important, too. Cats love treats, so encourage good behavior by rewarding him or her with a favorite goodie.

- Prefer a bird? Birds must have their cages cleaned every week. They also need to have their nails trimmed frequently.

- Favor a fish? Their vibrant colors are appealing, but their aquariums need to be cleaned regularly. That includes water treatments and new filters.

Tail-waggin' news: Cuddle that critter for a healthier heart, sounder sleep

"Dogs have a way of finding the people who need them, filling an emptiness we don't even know we have," said American author Thom Jones. Of course Jones only mentions dogs, but you probably feel the same way about your cat, rabbit, fish, bird, or any other animal you pick as a pet.

But besides filling that empty spot Jones mentions, researchers say owning pets may improve your blood pressure, cholesterol levels, and even your body's reaction to stress. Here are two ways your playful pooch can keep you healthy.

"Paws" a minute for better heart health. Just consider this. A Swedish study of nearly 337,000 folks who suffered either a stroke or heart attack found that those who owned a dog had a lower risk of dying after coming home from the hospital. Researchers say the reduced risk might be related to the increased physical activity that comes hand in paw with dog ownership. Having a dog at home also decreases depression and loneliness — and even lowers blood pressure, which is so important for maintaining a healthy brain.

Let sleeping dogs lie, and you will, too. Sleep, that is. According to a study of more than 6,500 seniors between the ages of 59 and 79, dog owners had less trouble falling asleep than people who didn't have dogs. Researchers think this may be because dog owners walk their dogs just before going to bed, and this could help them relax more easily and fall asleep more quickly. And according to the Centers for Disease Control and Prevention, a good night's sleep of at least seven hours is especially important for keeping blood pressure at normal levels and for staving off depression.

Paw-some ways to save big bucks on your pet

"How much is that doggie in the window? The one with the waggly tail?" Singer Patti Page made a hit out of this lighthearted song back in the 1950s. You can bet caring for that waggly-tailed pup will set you back a whole lot more today than it did back then.

When you add up the expense of adopting a pet — food, vet visits, grooming, and more — the average yearly cost for a dog ranges from $380 to $1,170. A cat will run you between $430 and $870. But you can keep cash in your wallet by checking with your state's Humane Society for financial assistance.

Talk to your vet about a payment plan if expensive treatments are needed. Or contact RedRover, an organization dedicated to helping animals in crisis, at *redrover.org*. Consider setting aside $1,000 just for medical emergencies.

Robotic seal brings comfort to seniors

There are robot lawn mowers. Robot vacuum cleaners. Even robot laundry folders. But robot pets? No way!

More than 60 seniors diagnosed with mild to moderate dementia were divided into control and treatment groups. Over three months, the treatment group was given the chance to spend 20 minutes three times each week with a new playful pal. It didn't seem to matter that this particular pal was a robot made to look like a furry, white seal.

In the group that interacted with the robot, research showed that the seal eased the seniors' symptoms of anxiety and depression, often in lieu of drugs. Improvement in pain — and less use of pain medications — were observed in this group, too.

Prayer

Rely on religion to bump up your brainpower

Spirituality and religion are an important part of many lives and often become even more so with age. That might make it a perfect time to become more active in the religious organization you belong to.

Along with building friendships, you'll likely see a host of health benefits. Researchers at Duke University found that African Americans and female seniors who engaged in religious activity like prayer and Bible reading were less likely than others to need care in nursing homes or rehab centers.

Want to combat cognitive decline? Try joining the church.

Studies suggest that people who go to church and pray regularly have slower rates of cognitive decline. Researchers think praying may help to strengthen the communication between nerve cells in your brain, train your memory, and improve your attention. And people who are involved in their church often have strong social networks, which may help keep sadness at bay.

Researchers tested that theory in a study of 64 seniors with Alzheimer's disease. The volunteers were tested on their cognitive abilities and sorted into two groups based on how religious they were.

A year later, the experts discovered that the seniors who reported being less religious experienced a faster rate of cognitive decline than those who were more religious. Moreover, the caregivers of the less-religious seniors also experienced more stress.

Pray away depression and anxiety. It should come as no surprise that prayers are a powerful balm for your troubles. A study published in *The International Journal of Psychiatry in Medicine* suggests that prayers can help blunt depression, anxiety, and other negative emotions.

Researchers recruited 63 adults with anxiety and depression and randomly assigned them to a control group or a prayer group. People in the prayer group met with a counselor, who guided them through weekly hourlong prayer sessions that focused on traumatic memories or other causes of emotional stress. In some cases, people used these six prayer sessions to ask for help in healing.

At the end of the study, people in the prayer group reported lower levels of depression and anxiety than a control group that didn't receive similar counseling. Researchers think the prayer intervention helped people deal with negative emotions that were tied to their past experiences. This, in turn, soothed their feelings of anxiety and depression.

Heal thyself — 2 ways faith fights high blood pressure and diabetes

People have long prayed for good health. Experts are now realizing there may be a solid, scientific reason for that. Research suggests that people who are more religious are better equipped to fend off high blood pressure and take control of type 2 diabetes.

Worried about high blood pressure? Your church may help lower your risk. Keeping your blood pressure under control is important, especially if you want to stay healthy as you age. High blood pressure is one of the most common causes of strokes and has long been linked with the development of Alzheimer's disease.

Fortunately, staying healthy could be as simple as getting more involved in your church.

In a large-scale study, American researchers polled 21,686 women about how religious or spiritual they were. They also recorded information about their blood pressure. After sifting through the data, the experts discovered that the women who used religion or spirituality to cope with stressful situations had a lower risk of hypertension.

The reason? The study's authors think religion may help people reduce stress, which is a major risk factor in developing high blood pressure.

Call on religion to help control type 2 diabetes. Managing blood sugar spikes is no easy feat if you have type 2 diabetes. But you need to stay on top of this disease because high glucose levels can damage your blood vessels, putting you at risk for vascular dementia. This decline in thinking skills is caused by reduced or blocked blood flow to the brain.

A new study in the *Journal of Marital and Family Therapy* suggests that managing your blood sugar could be easier if you and your spouse turn to religion to help cope with the challenge. Researchers looked at the religious habits of 87 couples in which one spouse had diabetes and the other didn't.

- They found that spouses without diabetes who viewed God as an ally in managing stress were more likely to share habits that helped their partner cope with the disease, such as planning healthy meals.

- And spouses with diabetes who felt abandoned by God because of their disease were less likely to share with their partner in good lifestyle choices that kept glucose levels under control.

> A fresh take on your prayer routine can help you feel a new enthusiasm and energy for your spiritual journey. Try praying under a large shady tree, in a garden, or by a lake. Or instead of sitting or kneeling while you pray, go for a short walk.

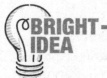

BRIGHT IDEA

Keep a journal to help strengthen your spiritual journey

Writing down what you're praying about is a powerful way to reflect on your blessings and confront your concerns. That's why many people keep prayer journals. If you don't think of yourself as a writer, don't worry. Here are four steps to start recording your spiritual journey.

- Decide how you're going to use your journal. Some people need a set structure of when and how they're going to pray. If that's you, decide on a time and place where you can sit and reflect with your prayer journal. But if you're more of a free spirit, simply carry your journal with you and write when a prayer comes into your mind.

- Use your journal to record the good moments. Every day, take the time to jot down three or four things that you're thankful for. Focusing on the blessings in your life — even small ones like a good night's sleep — can help you feel more grateful and positive.

- Don't ignore the bad moments. Your prayer journal is a great place to write down and reflect on concerns that you're dealing with. Some people suggest writing out a question to ponder every day. They can be big, broad questions or personal concerns like "Why am I not seeing eye to eye with my spouse about an issue?"

- Remember to go back through your journal. As you fill out a prayer journal, you should take time to write down when your prayers were made and if they have been answered. In the future, you can flip back through the pages and see how much you've grown spiritually.

Protein

Bulk up your diet to defend against brain damage

Proteins are key building blocks in your body. From your skin down to your bones, this nutrient helps you stay sharp and in shape. Find out how eating enough protein can keep your brain in tiptop condition.

Stop dementia before it starts. Scientists may not be able to cure Alzheimer's disease (AD) right now, but they do have a suggestion for prevention — eat enough protein to ward off the beta-amyloid plaques found in the brains of people with this type of dementia.

That's according to a study of 162 cognitively normal people over the age of 60 who provided details on their diets over the previous year. Researchers used that information to learn how many grams of protein the participants ate each day. They found that the people who ate the most protein were less likely to have large amounts of plaque in their brains.

Although more research is needed to fully understand the reason behind protein's impact, scientists suggest it may be linked to reduced blood pressure. That's important because high blood pressure is a risk factor for AD.

Protein beats back the blues. Food affects how you feel beyond calming hunger pangs and boosting energy levels. It can influence your emotions, too. For instance, experts believe your diet is related to your risk of depression.

Searching for more information about just that, a group of scientists gathered data from more than 75,000 adults who participated in national health and nutrition surveys. They found that people with diets lacking in protein had higher odds of depression than those who got normal amounts.

Strike a balance in your protein consumption

Goldilocks is known as a very particular, uninvited guest in the classic fairy tale "Goldilocks and the Three Bears." But when it comes to finding a happy medium, she may have been "just right." With protein you don't want to eat too much or too little.

A low-protein diet can lead to many serious conditions, including anemia and lowered immunity. That's why reaching your daily recommended goal of just over 7 grams for every 20 pounds of body weight is important. If you weigh 140 pounds, that's about 50 grams of protein every day.

How much protein you need may vary slightly from that calculated number depending on your activity level. People who engage in intense physical exercise need more.

Don't overdo it, though. Eating too much protein for a long time can lead to problems with your digestion, heart, and kidneys.

Meet your goal to avoid these 3 conditions

Growing up, your parents may have warned you to close your mouth or you'd catch flies. Insects may not be your top choice of a protein provider, but they're often more dense with this nutrient than familiar foods like beef and chicken. Whether you go the typical route or opt for something adventurous, getting enough protein is essential as you age.

This nutrient weighs in against weight gain. Obesity raises your risk of developing conditions linked to dementia, including heart disease and type 2 diabetes. According to researchers who reviewed 35 studies on the topic, protein may help you lose excess pounds.

The hormone leptin plays a critical role in controlling body weight, body fat mass, appetite, and the number of calories you burn. It may seem odd, but most people with obesity have higher leptin levels in their blood. Their condition may cause leptin resistance, meaning their bodies don't respond to this hormone anymore.

A possible remedy? Switching to a high-protein, low-calorie diet. Eating more protein may increase leptin concentration, sensitivity to leptin, and feelings of fullness — all of which can help with weight management.

Stave off stroke with a sea of protein. Strokes can be damaging within minutes, catastrophic within hours. Depending on what part of your brain is affected and for how long, your memory, motor skills, speech, behavior, and thought processes can become impaired.

But studies suggest protein can lessen your risk. Using data on over 250,000 people, researchers found that those who ate the most protein had a 20% lower risk of stroke than those who ate the least.

Don't compromise other aspects of your health in a bid to get more protein, though. Most animal proteins contain unhealthy fats. But fish like salmon, mackerel, and tuna are packed with good fats that help prevent blood clots and lower blood pressure. Beans, nuts, and dairy are other protein-rich options that won't increase your risk of heart disease, a risk factor for stroke.

Tip the scales against muscle loss the smart way. Age-related declines in muscle mass and function — a condition called sarcopenia — increase your risk of falls and frailty. Moreover, researchers have found that sarcopenia raises the odds of cognitive impairment and depression in seniors.

Because your muscles may process protein less efficiently as you age, eating enough of this nutrient is key to preventing this disease. "Older individuals need to eat more protein to get the same muscle-building response as younger and middle-aged

If you're trying to maximize your protein intake, preparation counts. Meats like beef and chicken lose protein under high heat. That's why low and slow is the way to go. A slow cooker set at low heat for a longer time will fully cook meat and ward off protein loss. For fish, try poaching or steaming.

people," says Dr. Benoit Smeuninx, an author of a study on protein and muscle loss published in *Frontiers in Nutrition*.

Seniors should also spread their protein consumption over the course of their day to maximize the benefits. Lunch is an especially good meal to increase your protein intake. The researchers found that older adults were more likely to eat bread at this meal. Young and middle-aged folks, on the other hand, ate more protein-rich foods like chicken and fish at lunch.

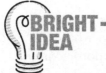

BRIGHT IDEA

No meat, no problem: Find the best plant proteins

Calling all vegetarians and omnivores! Peanuts and spinach may not be the first first food you think of when you hear "protein." But plant-based foods can help you achieve your daily goal — 46 grams (g) for the average woman and 56 g for the average man. The key is to eat a wide variety of them, rather than just your favorite one or two. That's because only a few sources of plant-based "complete proteins" exist.

Complete proteins provide you with all nine essential amino acids you must get through your diet. Soy and quinoa are two sources of complete proteins, but the vast majority of plant-based foods aren't. Eat a wide variety of them to get the nine amino acids your body can't make.

Try mixing these high-protein veggies into your meals to get all the amino acids you need.

Food	Protein (g) per cup
boiled lentils	17.9
boiled lima beans	11.6
fresh green peas	7.9
grilled portobello mushrooms	5.2
canned yellow sweet corn	5

Puzzles and games

Major win: Play your way to a brighter brain

The supervillain Riddler uses his obsession with riddles to devise criminal plots. Batman always thwarts his evil plans, but Riddler stays mentally sharp. He knows a thing or two about the brain benefits of puzzling.

Try board games to get your brain in gear. Working on mentally challenging activities could help protect your brain as you age, according to scientists in Japan. They surveyed 5,300 seniors and found better brain function in those who did activities like solving crossword puzzles and playing board games compared to those who didn't.

In fact, enjoying a little friendly competition is a good prescription for your mental health. Researchers learned that playing one of humanity's oldest board games — Go — can also improve your visual working memory, which relates to how you store and use visual information. They assigned seniors to a social group that interacted while playing Go, a solo group that used a tablet to play, or a control group.

Both game groups showed improvements in memory — with the social group getting slightly better scores — compared to the control. That may be because of the brain stimulation involved in recognizing, memorizing, and responding to their opponents' moves.

Puzzled about the best way to activate your mind? Think about how many times you have to turn jigsaw pieces to fit them in a puzzle. The odd shapes, colors, and patterns all have to match.

Putting them together requires mental flexibility and emotional control. So it should be no surprise that lifelong jigsaw puzzling may protect your brain. And it's relaxing to boot.

That's according to researchers who found more self-reported jigsaw puzzle experience over a lifetime was linked to better visual-spatial skills — the kind that help you readily tap into mental processes like reasoning and perception.

Keep your brain spry — work crosswords and sudoku. That's the advice coming from researchers in the PROTECT study — a 25-year online project tracking how often more than 19,000 seniors worked puzzles. Results show that regularly playing word and number puzzles keeps your brain working better for longer.

Not sure? Another finding from a 68-year study out of Scotland shows that playing more games like cards, chess, bingo, or crosswords is associated with higher cognitive function at age 70 and less cognitive decline, particularly in memory, from age 70 to 79. Plus participants who started playing more between 70 and 76 had less decline in cognitive speed — the ability to process information rapidly.

The findings support the "use it or lose it" hypothesis that putting your brain to work by playing games can help keep your noggin in fine fettle.

Fun and games restore well-being for folks living with dementia

Ever hosted a game night for family or friends? The spirited laughter and bonding that comes from playing together goes a long way toward creating a feeling of well-being. But forgetfulness and distraction can make people with mild cognitive impairment (MCI) — the stage between normal brain aging and dementia — wary of joining in such activities, leading to social isolation or depression. It doesn't have to be that way. Enter fun and games.

One study of seniors with MCI had participants play four games that required them to find, match, solve math problems, and complete pictures. The tasks required language, memory, attention, and spatial reasoning skills.

After playing these games developed specifically for people with MCI, participants reported positive feelings about their experiences. And researchers concluded that brain games can promote active aging — maintaining well-being as you age by staying engaged socially, mentally, and physically.

Researchers are working on ways to fine-tune games to make them even more helpful to people fighting MCI and dementia. But some games that show promise may already be in your cabinet.

- Bingo. It brings people together in friendly competition while it also asks you to pay close attention with your eyes and your ears. You have to use your fingers to place the tokens on your card so you're reinforcing fine motor skills. A game that stimulates the brain without being overwhelming for someone with dementia? Bingo!

- Mahjong. In this game you have to pay attention to the tiles your opponent has played in order to predict their upcoming moves and build your strategy to win. When seniors with MCI played this game at least three hours a week for three months as part of a study they saw improvements in executive function, their ability to regulate their own behavior, pay attention, organize, and achieve goals.

- Call to mind. Developed by an occupational therapist specifically for people with dementia, this game gets folks talking about their experiences and opinions. They interact with a game board and each other as they share memories.

Hungarian chess player Janos Flesch set a record for blindfolded chess in 1960. He played 52 opponents at once and managed to win 31 games. That's even more amazing when you consider you have over nine million positions available to you after both players make their first three moves.

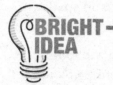 **BRIGHT IDEA**

Free ways to challenge your brain online

Are you tempted to pay for an app that claims it will make you smarter? Save your money. Lots of apps offer ample opportunity to exercise your brain — all for free. Look for these games that you can get from the app store on Android or iPhone.

- NeuroNation. Picked as an Editors' Choice by the Google Play Store, this app starts with a few questions so it can map out the best experience for you. After an "assessment" round for practice, you may choose the pathfinder exercise or take a different route tailored to your specifications. You can play three games for free daily.

- WordBrain. At first, you might think WordBrain's tantalizing puzzles are child's play, but don't be fooled. These clever word puzzles start off easy and get harder.

- Tricky Test 2: Genius Brain. Like brain teasers? This app is full of clever questions that will keep you challenged, entertained, and amused.

- Brain It On. If you like shapes, look no further than this physics-inspired puzzle game. Play solo or with friends to solve each puzzle.

- Two Dots. Artists will love the minimalist design on this award-winning puzzle where you connect and match dots to master challenges.

- Jigsaw Puzzles Real. Play on the go. Choose from 2,400 photos ranging from novice to expert difficulty. Or create a jigsaw out of a photo from your own digital gallery.

- Move the Block: Slide Puzzle. Test your spatial reasoning skills by moving the red block through a maze of other blocks to get to the exit. Try to solve it without hints.

Quercetin

Know your onions — this powerful pigment gives your mind some extra might

Onions used to be so prized in the Middle Ages that people would give them as gifts. While opening up a birthday present only to find a few onions might not sound great, there's a good reason to get excited about them. These bulbous vegetables, particularly the red and yellow varieties, are some of the best sources of quercetin — a naturally occurring pigment that can help boost your brainpower.

Maximize your memory with a heaping helping of quercetin. As you get older, you might realize your powers of recall aren't exactly what they used to be. Fortunately, getting more quercetin may help jog your memory.

In a small study, seniors with Alzheimer's disease completed memory tests before and after taking a quercetin-rich onion powder daily for four weeks. Then they took a monthlong break before repeating the experiment with an onion powder made from white onions, which are low in quercetin.

At the end of the study, researchers found that the quercetin-rich supplement was linked with greater improvements in memory compared to the other onion powder. The study authors think quercetin may work by improving the processes in your brain involved with recalling memories.

If you want to try this yourself, seniors in the study got 80 milligrams (mg) of quercetin each day. On average, you'd have to eat almost two red onions to get that amount through your diet. But keep in mind, the quercetin content of onions can vary widely depending on the variety and growing conditions. It's no surprise then that many people turn to supplements.

These pungent plants will help keep your brain from aging.
Don't skip out on onions just because you're afraid of bad breath. New research published in *Functional Foods in Health and Disease* suggests the quercetin in onions can help keep your brain young.

Researchers recruited 50 seniors and asked them to take onion powder every day. Some were given a powder that contained 60 mg of quercetin, while the others were given a placebo powder.

After 24 weeks, researchers found that the seniors who received quercetin showed slower rates of cognitive decline than the control group.

3 ways quercetin can protect your heart

Avoiding heart disease is a key part of keeping your brain healthy. Risk factors for cardiovascular disease — such as high blood pressure, obesity, and cholesterol — can all contribute to stroke, dementia, and even memory problems. Luckily, one little nutrient may help you keep all three of these conditions in check.

Battle high blood pressure with this simple supplement.
High blood pressure is one of the most common causes of strokes and has long been linked with the development of Alzheimer's disease. So if you want to stay healthy as you age, keeping those numbers down is important.

There's good news, though. Experts say quercetin may help do the trick. An analysis published in the *Journal of the American Heart Association* examined

Looking into quercetin supplements? Some research suggests that high doses — think 500 to 1,000 milligrams a day — could cause headaches, nausea, and an upset stomach. Use caution if you're already taking medications to lower your blood pressure. And talk to your doctor before adding any new supplements.

seven studies that included a total of 587 participants. The authors concluded that getting more than 500 milligrams (mg) of quercetin from supplements every day was linked with a drop in blood pressure.

The reason? Experts think quercetin may help fight off inflammation and oxidative stress associated with high blood pressure.

Getting the study-recommended dose through your diet alone would be a steep challenge. But the authors suggest that supplements might be a good add-on to a treatment plan for high blood pressure, and they call for more trials.

Do you want to lose weight and melt away fat? Bring on the quercetin. Carrying around too much extra weight can wreak havoc on your health. Obesity — and the heart disease and diabetes that often accompany it — could damage your blood vessels and disrupt the flow of oxygen-rich blood to your brain. Fortunately, a bit of quercetin can help you slim down.

Researchers from South Korea recruited 72 overweight adults and split them up into two groups. Half were asked to take 100 mg of quercetin daily in the form of an onion peel extract, while the other half were given a placebo. Then, after three months, researchers checked in to see who had lost the most weight.

They found that the quercetin group dropped more pounds than people on the placebo. Even better? They lost significant amounts of body fat, too.

Say goodbye to high cholesterol with quercetin. When your arteries and blood vessels become clogged with cholesterol, your brain doesn't get enough oxygen. Brain cells begin to die and you experience problems like short-term memory loss. But a recent meta-analysis found quercetin may help put an end to those worries.

The new study, published in the journal *Critical Reviews in Food Science and Nutrition*, examined 16 studies about the effects of quercetin on cholesterol. The paper revealed that quercetin helps decrease total levels of cholesterol and LDL — or "bad" — cholesterol.

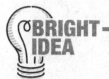

Want to get more quercetin? Use these top tips

Nutrition labels won't tell you how much quercetin is in your meals. Here's a handy list to see which foods pack the most milligrams (mg).

Food	Quercetin (mg) per serving
red onion	43.1
yellow onion	22.3
capers	18.7
kale	15.1
apple, with skin	6.9
white onion	6.8
broccoli	3
scallions	2.7

Choosing quercetin-rich foods isn't the only way to get more of this powerful nutrient. Try these simple tips, too.

- Pair quercetin with fiber for a one-two punch. Research suggests that your body can absorb more quercetin when you eat it with insoluble fiber, like the kind you'd find in whole-grain breads or wheat bran.

- Don't be afraid of a bit of fat. You can also get more quercetin from your foods when you eat them with fats. Try adding a drizzle of oil to a kale and onion salad. Just make sure to opt for healthier choices, like olive oil or canola oil, instead of butter.

- Save your onion skins to get more nutrients. The papery, outer layer of onions are chock-full of quercetin, but they're not easy to eat. Simply simmer them into a stock or stew and strain them out before you dig in.

Reading and learning

3 ways to keep your brain sharp into your 90s

At 105 years old, retired Maj. Bill White holds the title of the oldest living Marine. His secret to a long life? It's not physical exercise. Instead, he claims reading regularly helps him keep his mind in tiptop shape. And research suggests the decorated World War II veteran has a point.

Want to dodge dementia? Crack open a book. Every year, nearly 10 million people develop dementia worldwide. If you don't want to count yourself among them, you need to keep your mind active. And researchers think reading may be a great way to do just that.

In a recent study published in *JAMA Psychology*, researchers polled 15,582 seniors about their hobbies and leisure activities. Then they kept tabs on these people for five years. The study revealed that those who spent time doing mentally stimulating hobbies — like reading — were less likely to develop dementia.

The reason? Experts think reading may improve your cognitive reserve, which means your brain is more resistant to the damage caused by dementia. Plus spending more time reading helps beef up the parts of your brain involved with memory and learning.

You can give your social skills a boost by escaping into fiction. Keeping your social skills sharp can help prevent the harmful effects of age-related memory loss. And a study conducted by researchers at Harvard University reveals that reading fiction may help people connect with others.

In a small study, researchers asked people to read sections of books, newspapers, and magazines while undergoing an MRI. The scans showed that those who regularly read fiction had more activity in specific areas of the brain when reading about people. The scientists say this may translate into improved social skills by exercising those parts of the brain associated with empathy and imagination.

Reading helps soothe stress. Need to decompress after a long day? Research shows that sitting down with a good book could be exactly what you need.

A study conducted by American researchers tested the stress-relieving powers of reading against two other pastimes. Participants were divided into three groups and asked to spend 30 minutes once a week reading articles about history and technology, doing yoga, or watching comedy videos. At the end of each of three weekly sessions, all three groups saw reductions in their heart rates, blood pressure, and stress levels.

The study's authors also point out that the reading group found the half hour of reading to be relaxing. The scientists say that reading may help relax the sympathetic nervous system, which reduces overall feelings of stress. So if your book or newspaper makes you feel anxious, put it down and read something soothing instead.

> If you or someone you know has trouble reading due to vision loss, don't worry. The National Library Service offers free talking books and braille books for people with vision problems. Check with your local library. Or go online to *loc.gov/nls* or call 888-NLS-READ to find out more.

Love to learn? Continuing education can save your brain

A garden can't flourish on its own. You need to water your plants, pluck the weeds, and put fertilizer in the soil. And something similar is true for your mind. Research shows that learning can help you make a natural "brain fertilizer" — known as brain-derived neurotrophic factor — which boosts blood flow and neural connections in the brain. Here are a few other ways learning slows cognitive decline.

Keep your mind sharp by heading back to the classroom.
Thought your school days were behind you? You might want to think again. New research suggests that taking adult education classes can help keep your brain younger.

Irish researchers recently published a paper in the *International Journal of Geriatric Psychiatry* that looked at how late-in-life education impacts the minds of seniors. They recruited 5,306 people and asked them about the levels of education they had achieved and if they had taken any adult education classes in the past year.

The study revealed that the people who took continuing education courses had better overall cognitive function than those who didn't. The authors aren't exactly sure why, but they think late-in-life studies help improve the brain's resistance to age-related damage. And as an added benefit, classes helped the seniors stay more socially engaged.

Learning another language bolsters your brainpower. Ever dream of dining on the banks of the Seine? You might need to brush up on your French. Planning to visit the Great Wall of China? It's time to start practicing your Mandarin. Even if you're not planning a grand adventure, you might want to spend some time learning another language.

Researchers polled 853 seniors about how many languages they spoke, how often they spoke a second language, and what age they were when they learned it. The seniors then underwent a series of memory, verbal, and general intelligence tests designed to examine their brainpower.

The results revealed that the seniors who spoke more than one language had better-than-expected cognitive abilities for people of their age, even if they didn't learn another language until they were adults. The researchers think speaking two or more languages improves executive function. Those are the skills you need to pay attention, plan and organize, and remember small details.

BRIGHT IDEA

Top tips to help you get back to school

Ready to hit the books again? With a little know-how, you can find cheap — or even free — classes if you're a senior.

- Become a senior scholar for free. Why not sign up for continuing education classes at your local public college? Classes are often free or discounted for adults age 60 and above. Go to *aseniorcitizenguideforcollege.com* and click on "Find Your State Tuition Waivers" in the menu at the top of the page.

- Ask your local college if you can audit a class. You won't get a grade or credit, but you'll definitely boost your knowledge. You also could try shorter-term classes offered through local community centers and libraries.

- Don't forget about financial aid. Government programs and independent organizations often give scholarships to seniors who want to return to school. Call up the college or university you want to attend and ask them about any grants or scholarship offers.

- Head to the web to learn in the comfort of your own home. Can't find any classes at your local college that interest you? The internet boasts thousands of hours of courses, with topics that range from physics to Beethoven. You can find free classes from top-notch schools like Harvard University and the University of California, Berkeley at *edx.org*. Stanford University offers courses at *online.stanford.edu/free-courses*.

Sauna

Sweat the big stuff to dry up your dementia risk

Can you think of a room in your home that could be used for just about anything? For people in Finland, that space would be the sauna. Today they bathe there to relieve stress. But traditionally they also used it for birthing babies, curing meat, and many other activities.

Most Fins practice sauna bathing weekly — and even in the U.S. people are beginning to adopt the ritual. Why? Aside from its soothing effects, users swear by a cleansing sauna bath's other health benefits.

Saunas use dry heat, unlike steam baths that offer high humidity. Traditional saunas look like closets with bench seating and can be heated by burning wood, electricity, or infrared heat. You may also find water for pouring over hot rocks to create steam.

Science suggests that dry heat has benefits for the mind. In fact, regular sauna bathing was associated with a lower risk of dementia in men. Researchers followed 2,315 healthy Finnish men for 20 years. The men who reported taking a sauna two to seven times per week were less likely to develop dementia or Alzheimer's disease compared to those who took one sauna bath a week.

What makes saunas effective for your brain? Experts say sauna bathing may improve blood pressure and blood vessel function, which in turn can lower your risk for dementia.

Heat therapy helps make healthier hearts and minds

Imagine relaxing in a hot sauna room, tension seeping out of your body with each droplet of perspiration. Halfway through a yawn, the door swings open and a Finnish woman approaches you, wash bucket in hand, ready to scrub you down.

If you weren't expecting this Finnish tradition, your blood pressure might shoot back up. But don't fret — the Finnish washing lady only makes appearances in saunas in Finland. What you should expect from regular sauna bathing would be the same benefits for your heart, mind, and blood vessels that Fins experience.

Inside the sauna, heat drives up your heart rate and causes your blood vessels to widen. This improves circulation much like low to moderate exercise. It may help your heart and mind in three ways.

- **Slash your stroke risk.** Out of 1,628 Finnish adults in one study, those who visited the sauna four to seven times per week over 15 years had a much lower risk of having a stroke compared to those who took only one sauna bath a week.

- **Level high blood pressure.** Another study showed that after a 30-minute sauna bath, participants' blood pressure dropped seven points and remained lower than pre-sauna levels even half an hour later.

> Make the most of your relaxing getaway in a sauna by taking focused, deep breaths. Add in the pleasant aromas of essential oils and the soothing sounds of calming music for your own personalized spa experience.

- **Hamper heart disease.** Researchers who studied Finnish seniors found that those who took four to seven sauna baths a week had a lower risk of dying from heart disease over a 14-year period. The risk was also less for those who spent more than 45 minutes per week in a sauna.

The blood vessel damage involved in these three conditions can pave the way for brain problems. Luckily, frequent trips to the sauna may take the heat off those worries. Hot ziggety!

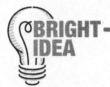

Hot tips: Sauna safely for the best experience

Did you know you can lose a pint of sweat while sauna bathing? That's why you should drink plenty of water — like two to four glasses — before and after your experience. It'll help you avoid dehydrating. Surprised? Here are more tips to make sure your experience is helpful and healthy.

- Step in clean and light. Most sauna bathers advise a quick rinse before sitting in the heat. Avoid alcohol and a heavy meal. Take off your jewelry and cosmetic products. Wear loose-fitting, clean clothing without any metal — if you wear anything at all.

- Sweat it out safely. Sweat helps your body cool down, but as you get older, your body sweats less and you're more prone to heat-related health issues. If you're new to saunas, sit on the lowest seat where the heat is less intense. Limit your visit time to five to 10 minutes. Once you get used to the sauna, you can stay up to 20 minutes.

- Consider Finnish-ing touches. The Fins tap their skin with birch twigs in the sauna. They claim it increases blood circulation and speeds up perspiration. And they like how it smells. Some like to wrap up their sauna with a shower or a quick swim to cool down.

- Sidestep serious sauna no-nos. Talk to your doctor before stepping in a sauna if you use a medical device, such as a pacemaker or defibrillator, or have health concerns like kidney disease, low blood pressure, or heart conditions. Saunas may compound the effects of medications that make you drowsy, impair your judgment, or affect your ability to sweat.

Sleep

Kip down for the night and skip memory loss

Once upon a time you fell asleep as soon as your head hit the pillow. Now your story is more "The Princess and the Pea" than "Sleeping Beauty." An errant legume is just one reason you may be sleeping poorly. Health conditions like allergies, arthritis, and anxiety as well as certain meds can make it tough to catch your ZZZs.

But you have good reason to aim for sweeter slumber. In fact, slowing down mental aging may be as simple as getting enough sleep.

Maximize your memory with a night's rest. Don't scrimp on sleep if you want to keep your memory sharp as a tack. Research shows taking a snooze can help your memory recall.

In one such study, participants were quizzed on their memories of made-up words right after learning them. They were tested a second time after either a night of sleep or a period of daytime wakefulness. The people who slept were more likely to remember words they'd previously known and missed.

"Sleep almost doubles our chances of remembering previously unrecalled material," says researcher Nicolas Dumay of the University of Exeter. "The post-sleep boost in memory accessibility may indicate that some memories are sharpened overnight. This supports the notion that, while asleep, we actively rehearse information flagged as important."

And that's why getting enough rest is the secret to staying mentally alert as you age.

Doze off to diminish dementia. Avoiding dementia doesn't have to be a far-fetched fantasy. Rapid-eye movement (REM) sleep is when most dreaming occurs, and not getting enough is tied to dementia.

REM sleep features high levels of brain activity. Scientists theorize that this activity protects connections in your brain that are susceptible to damage as you age. In one study, researchers found that people over 60 who spent less time in REM sleep were more likely to develop dementia over a 12-year span than those who had gotten more.

Lighten your blues when you snooze. If you find yourself waking up in the middle of the night or feeling down during the day, you're not alone. Interrupted sleep and depression are two of the most common symptoms of insomnia.

That's especially important because studies suggest disruptions in your sleeping pattern can raise your risk of depression. One influential change is a drop in slow wave sleep (SWS) — also called deep sleep. In one study, researchers found that people woken up multiple times during the night showed decreases in positive mood and increases in negative mood compared to those who slept a full night undisturbed.

Interestingly, some researchers suggest that a loss of SWS may affect the process where your brain converts positive emotional short-term memories into long-term ones.

Newer research shows deep sleep helps with other aspects of mood, too. "We have identified a new function of deep sleep, one that decreases anxiety overnight by reorganizing connections in the brain," says Matthew Walker, a University of California, Berkeley professor of neuroscience and psychology and senior author of a new study that reveals deep sleep may help your anxious brain. "Deep sleep seems to be a natural anxiolytic (anxiety inhibitor), so long as we get it each and every night."

You may need nine hours of sleep to feel bright-eyed and bushy-tailed when your partner feels wide awake after just six. Everyone's sleep needs vary, but research suggests between six and eight hours each night is the sweet spot for stroke protection. Consistently getting more or less shut-eye could put you at a greater risk.

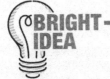

1 sheep, 2 sheep, 5 steps to a perfect night's sleep

Make your bedtime routine super simple with these tips. You can get the best rest you've had in ages when you do, eat, and drink these things before bed.

A melatonin-based bite is key to unlocking dreamland. Tart cherry juice and nuts are the perfect evening snack to reduce insomnia. Both contain high amounts of the hormone melatonin which experts believe helps promote sleepiness at night and wakefulness during the daytime. Don't drink too much, though. You don't want to wake up to go to the bathroom.

Wind down from your day before hitting the hay. Start getting in the sleep mindset one or two hours ahead of time. Try creating a quiet, restful environment, and add relaxing activities like reading a book to your nightly routine.

For better shut-eye, use a weighted blanket. Researchers think it's the comforting touch pressure of weighted blankets that helps people settle down and experience better quality sleep. Choose one that's about 10% of your body weight.

To drift off faster, find your happy place. Imagine a relaxing scene — like a mountain stream or a sunny beach — and concentrate on that instead of your everyday worries and concerns. Research shows you could fall asleep 20 minutes faster using this process called imagery distraction.

Keep a schedule for better sleep. Train your brain to differentiate between bedtime and wake-up call by keeping your meal and sleep times consistent.

Rest up to restore health across your body

Burning the midnight oil again? You may call it quits when you hear a lack of sleep can harm your overall health. Forty winks aren't enough to keep your ability to think, focus, react, and learn up to snuff.

And the effects of sleep stretch far and wide — influencing your heart, weight, blood sugar, and immune system. Problems in those areas can damage blood vessels, disrupt blood flow, and cause other changes that may circle back and harm your brain. Find out how sleep may be the source of your troubles.

- Heart. While you sleep your body is busy at work repairing your heart and blood vessels. Make the most of this unconscious healing time by not sleeping too much or too little. You'll also help keep a balance of stress hormones that play a role in cardiovascular disease.

- Weight. Sleep loss may leave you too tired to exercise. But physical fitness isn't the only factor in weight gain. Sleep helps keep your hunger hormones, ghrelin and leptin, in check. Leptin levels, which control feelings of fullness, go down when you're behind on sleep. And ghrelin, which makes you feel hungry, goes up.

- Blood sugar. Insulin is the hormone in charge of your blood sugar level. Research suggests that sleep impacts your body's reaction to insulin. Staying up to the wee hours of the night can make your cells more resistant to insulin and lead to higher blood sugar levels.

- Immune system. You may feel sick more often if you don't get enough quality sleep. That's because when you sleep your immune system releases helpful proteins — some of which help your body respond to infection and inflammation. Without them your body's defenses may go down.

Wake-up call: Think twice before you take sleeping pills

Popping a pill before you hit the hay may seem like an easy way to head off your sleep troubles. But the nighttime fix that seems so simple may bring on serious consequences in the light of day.

"Although sleep problems can happen at any age and for many reasons, they can't be cured by taking a pill, either prescription, over-the-counter, or herbal, no matter what the ads on TV claim," says Preeti Malani, M.D., a University of Michigan physician trained in geriatric medicine. "Some of these medications can create big concerns for older adults, from falls and memory issues to confusion and constipation."

Over-the-counter sleep aids can cause a nightmare of side effects. Blurred vision, low blood pressure upon standing, dizziness, and heart palpitations. Just a few of the serious side effects linked to the antihistamines found in sleep medicines like Benadryl, Aleve PM, and Unisom SleepTabs.

These drugs sold over the counter at your local pharmacy may also interact with other medications you're taking. Check with your doctor or pharmacist for more information.

Don't fall for these prescription pills. Some prescription sleeping aids — like Xanax, Valium, and Restoril — contain benzodiazepines, man-made medications that help you get to sleep by upping the effects of GABA neurotransmitters that slow down brain activity.

But the use of benzodiazepines has been linked with an increased risk of falls. Other side effects of benzodiazepines can include lightheadedness, confusion, nausea, and memory loss.

Try the natural alternative. The American Academy of Sleep Medicine recommends cognitive behavioral therapy (CBT) for folks suffering from chronic insomnia.

CBT involves regular visits with a clinician who will give you a series of sleep assessments. He will ask you to keep track of your sleep in a special diary. And he'll help you find ways to improve your sleep habits.

A recent study released by the Agency for Healthcare Research and Quality shows that even after therapy ends, CBT might keep those sleepless nights at bay longer than sleeping meds — with no scary side effects to worry about.

Out like a light — block the blues for a better snooze

Want better sleep? Turn off your e-reader. One study showed that people who read e-books before bedtime took 10 minutes longer to fall asleep than when they read paper books. Readers of e-books also felt less alert the following morning.

Scientists say the trouble is caused by blue light — emitted from devices like your e-reader, tablet, cellphone, computer, and flat-screen TV — which throws off your sleep cycle. So limit screen time two to three hours before snooze time.

Can't avoid your gadgets at night? Researchers recently discovered that when people wore blue light-blocking glasses for three hours before bedtime for two weeks, their nighttime levels of the sleep-regulating chemical melatonin increased by 58%. That's even better than the results you might get by taking over-the-counter melatonin supplements.

Don't lose sleep over breathless nights

Oh, the snoring. You've poked and prodded, tickled and tapped. You've tried earplugs. You're even thinking about making a move to the guest room for just one night of peaceful, uninterrupted shut-eye.

The problem? Your spouse has obstructive sleep apnea (OSA).

"Sleep apnea is worse than just snoring," says Dr. Nitun Verma, spokesperson for the American Academy of Sleep Medicine. "When a person's airway closes down completely, no air is moving, and oxygen levels start to drop." And that's when OSA puts you at risk for developing serious conditions like high blood pressure and diabetes. The lack of oxygen reaching your tissues may even increase your risk of Alzheimer's disease.

Two to three times as many men as women have OSA, but sometimes women slip through the gap because they have different symptoms. While men usually show signs like loud snoring and gasping for air, women are more likely to complain about depression, fatigue, and restless legs.

But men and women share the same health risks if the condition goes untreated, says Verma.

While sleep apnea can be controlled with lifestyle changes, like maintaining a healthy weight and limiting alcohol, doctors continue to recommend a CPAP machine — short for continuous positive airway pressure.

"CPAP is a successful treatment," says Verma. "However, it's not always a love-at-first-sight solution. On average it takes people two to six weeks to adjust."

If your mask is uncomfortable, Verma recommends talking to your doctor. "A better mask can make a world of difference," he says.

Shape up to slumber soundly

Getting enough physical activity during the day is your fast pass to a good night's sleep — no strict exercise routine required. For a restful night, experts say any energy spending movement will do.

Using up your energy through physical activity is related to better sleep efficiency, the amount of time you actually spend asleep while in bed. And higher sleep efficiency is associated with improvement in executive control processes including task switching and memory.

And that's not all. Research also suggests physical activity can improve sleep quality and brain function in seniors with mild cognitive impairment, the stage between normal brain aging and the more serious decline of dementia.

So grab your tennis shoes and embrace the benefits of counting reps instead of sheep.

Socialization

Hang out with your gang for a healthier brain and a happier life

Hester Ford of Charlotte, NC, has lived a long life. In fact, there will be 117 candles on her birthday cake next time around. Her secret for a long life? Her family believes it's her passion and love for friends and family that keep her going. "She just loved her people, she didn't allow them to be sick or hungry," her daughter Daisy Davis says.

And research shows that folks who are involved in meaningful activities with others have a sense of purpose. Such activities seem to help them maintain their well-being, and even improve their brainpower.

A sharper brain? That's what friends are for. Older adults with larger social networks show greater global cognitive function — that includes memory, learning, decision-making, and language — and a lower rate of cognitive decline as they age, according to a study of more than 6,000 seniors.

But don't worry, loners. Separate research suggests that older folks who live alone are at no greater risk for developing poor cognitive function than those who live with others. It's the social isolation that you've got to keep an eye on. Another reason to keep in touch with friends and family.

And believe this. Scientists examining data on nearly 17,000 seniors found that the rate of memory decline effectively doubles in the most socially isolated people compared with those who have the most social interaction.

Beat depression with a little help from your friends. The key to avoiding depression seems to be connecting with the right social group for you. Not just anyone will do.

In one study, people diagnosed with depression or anxiety joined either a community group with activities like sewing and yoga, or participated in group therapy. Of those who developed a strong connection to their group, less than a third still met the criteria for clinical depression a month later. Participants in both the community and therapy groups said the other members made them feel supported, as if they were all in it together.

"We were able to find clear evidence that joining groups, and coming to identify with them, can alleviate depression," says study author and University of Queensland professor of psychology Alexander Haslam.

Head off depression by staying in touch

Those regular Sunday visits to Grandma's house are doing more for her health than you think. A two-year study of 11,000 seniors showed that those who met often with family and friends were less likely to develop symptoms of depression than those who didn't.

In fact, study participants who had in-person visits at least three times per week had a 6.5% chance of having symptoms of depression. That rose to 11.5% in the people who saw loved ones once every few months or less. Friends and relatives live far away? No worries. A separate study found that seniors who kept in touch via video chat — like Skype — had about half the risk of depressive symptoms compared to nonusers and those who relied on email, social media, and instant messaging.

Tweets, pics, and posts: Seniors click safely on social media

Imagine this. A woman phones her grandson for some tech help. "What kind of computer do you have, Grandma?" She hesitates before answering, "A white one?" All joking aside, seniors have come a long way since the dawn of the internet decades ago. Even though only 40% of Americans over age 65 say they visit social media sites, that's a considerable jump from just a few years ago.

Are you thinking about trying out Twitter or Facebook? Maybe YouTube and Instagram have caught your eye. Just make sure you know social media's pros and cons before you post that first pic or tweet that first tweet.

"Liking" loved ones keeps them close — and makes you happy. Researchers found that people who interacted with friends and family members on Facebook showed increased levels of well-being, happiness, and satisfaction with life. Measures of loneliness and depression improved, as well.

Social media sites may increase your feelings of self-worth, too. Feeling a little down on yourself? Since users most often post pictures of happy times, take a stroll through your profile page. Look at all the things that are going well in your life. Those pictures and comments can really lift your spirits.

Don't get trapped in the net. Being safe online is mostly common sense. Just be sure to choose your online friends carefully. The old saying you learned as a child, "Don't talk to strangers," still applies. And never post private information like your address, birthday, or Social Security number.

> What kind of activities most interest seniors? The website *after55.com* says the top pick is yoga and exercise classes. No. 2 is walking and hiking. Water aerobics and swimming take third. What's at the bottom of the list? That well-known old-timer, shuffleboard. Guess it's time to shuffle on off to Buffalo, shuffleboard.

Keep an eye out for scams, too. Cyberthieves may try to steal your credit card information or capture your login and password credentials. If an unexpected ad or unusual message appears in one of your accounts, think before you click. If you're concerned about anything you see online, get advice from a trusted friend or family member.

This natural remedy racks up a hat trick of health benefits

The one change in your routine that can lower your blood pressure, fight loneliness, and even help manage your weight? Invest some time and effort into building a supportive community of friends and family.

Friends ease loneliness and lower your blood pressure. A study of nearly 230 seniors found that those who described themselves as lonely had blood pressure readings up to 30 points higher than those who had stronger social connections.

"Lonely people differ from nonlonely individuals in their tendency to perceive stressful circumstances as threatening rather than challenging," said John Cacioppo, an author of the study and a former professor of psychology at the University of Chicago. He explained that when lonely people try to cope with stress, they often fail to ask for emotional support. They often withdraw from stress rather than meeting their problems head-on.

Cacioppo's previous research found that stress increased resistance to blood flow in young adults, which can cause higher blood pressure over the lifetime of lonely people. In fact, a separate study published in the *Proceedings of the National Academy of Sciences* found that social isolation increased seniors' risk of high blood pressure more than diabetes, a more commonly known risk factor.

Manage your weight with a strong community network. Besides helping to manage your blood pressure — which can lead to brain problems like stroke — social interactions have been shown to reduce your chance of developing obesity as you grow older, according to researchers.

Bottom line? Older adults live longer if they have stronger social connections. So get in touch with an old friend, invite a neighbor for a walk, or ask the grandkids to pop over for movie night. Want to meet new people? Joining a book club is a fantastic way to make some friends.

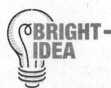

BRIGHT IDEA

Back up your brain with a strong social network

"People, people who need people, are the luckiest people in the world," sang Barbra Streisand in the 1964 Broadway musical, "Funny Girl." The wisdom in these words? Health and happiness hinge on folks making connections with each other. Research shows that your physical, cognitive, and emotional health require a good, solid social network of supportive people. But how do you find these people, people who need people, just like you?

Thrive with group hobbies. Do you like to knit, garden, or play chess? Perhaps you love to read or watch films. Either way, lots of clubs cater to a particular hobby.

Go to *meetup.com* or your local senior center to find groups with similar interests. Researchers have found that older seniors who are social and participate in arts and crafts run a reduced risk of developing dementia. While the data doesn't prove cause and effect, it can't hurt to have fun with people who have similar interests.

Build your network with healthy eating. Seniors, particularly those living alone, often don't eat enough or turn to prepackaged or frozen foods. After all, few people go to the trouble of cooking a big, healthy meal for just one person.

So it should come as no surprise that seniors say they are happier, enjoy the taste of food, and get more nutrition when sharing meals. Fortunately, finding a table mate is easier than you think. Why not invite a neighbor over for lunch or dinner? Better yet, go shopping and cook together. Your guest will most likely be grateful for your company.

Dial up newfound friends at a nationwide social center

Want to socialize with others from the comfort of your own home? Get in touch with Well Connected, a nonprofit that offers classes, friendly conversation, and support groups to older adults across the country. Once you register, you can access any of its 70 activities a week via conference call.

All you need is a telephone to take part in the free service. You can also use your computer to join online groups. On average, each group has about 12 participants. Well Connected will even set up reminder calls so you don't forget to dial in.

> Your sense of smell is the only one of your five senses directly linked to the limbic system, the parts of your brain that deal with emotions, instincts, and memory. That's why familiar scents — like your mother's soft perfume or freshly cut grass — can remind you of a pleasant experience and change your mood for the better.

"You can learn a foreign language, study art history, listen to poetry, play bingo, or be an armchair traveler — all over the phone," says Audrey Demmitt, a peer advisor for VisionAware, an organization dedicated to helping adults with vision loss stay independent. "It's a really great support network."

For more information, call 877-797-7299 toll free, or go online to *covia.org/services/well-connected*.

Soy

Lean on a better bean to face menopause

Soybeans are nutritious legumes that come from the pea family and may be the most widely used beans in the world. In fact, you can find soy and soybean oil in everything from burgers and animal feed to car tires and candles. Don't miss out on this tasty treat to keep your brain and body working at their best — even during the change of life.

Grab another helping of soybeans and cut your risk of cognitive decline. That's according to a study in Japan where women who reported regularly eating foods like soybeans, tofu, soy sauce, and miso experienced a lower risk of cognitive impairment over an average of almost eight years.

Soy products are chock-full of compounds called isoflavones. Inside your body, they behave like the hormone estrogen. Since women in phases of menopause have declining estrogen levels, they could benefit from eating soy foods. Experts suspect that isoflavones act through the central nervous system, which has its own estrogen receptors, to impact learning and memory.

Manage your menopause symptoms. There's nothing like a hot flash to amp up your anxiety, distract you from daily activities, or interrupt brain-replenishing sleep. But how can soy help? Researchers have spilled the beans.

Some of the physically uncomfortable side effects that occur in menopause — like hot flashes and night sweats — result from women's lower levels of estrogen. But because of isoflavones, soy may be a natural way to get the estrogen you need after menopause without hormone replacement therapy.

But not all women see benefits. Why? Studies have shown that only some women can convert soy isoflavones into an even more beneficial compound called equol. Researchers believe equol helps protect against the usual menopausal symptoms, as well as brittle bones and aging skin. Your body's ability to convert soy isoflavones to equol could make a huge difference in your results.

Put the pep back in your post-menopausal step. You might find renewed vigor from a compound called lecithin found mainly in egg yolks and soybeans.

Researchers in one study asked 89 middle-aged Japanese women who reported fatigue to take soy lecithin. Participants took either a high dose, low dose, or placebo as a supplement after breakfast daily.

At the end of eight weeks, women in the high-dose group reported more energy, and they showed improvement in risk factors for cardiovascular disease compared to the placebo group.

> Skip the additives and make your own soy milk. Rinse and soak 1/2 cup of soybeans in 2 to 3 cups of water overnight. Blend them in the water, then strain with a fine-woven cheesecloth. Heat the mixture on low for 20 minutes, stirring often. Allow the milk to cool before storing in the fridge.

You'll be soy amazed at 2 ways this little legume helps your health

Here's a grocery hack you might like. Keep roasted soybeans on hand in case you run low on java. Grind them up coarsely and treat them like you would regular coffee grounds. Soy coffee brews up a number of perks — it's easy to make, caffeine-free, cheap, and healthy. In fact, you might find other soy foods keep you in fine feather, too.

Turn to new flavors to score better sleep. Tofu, made from soybean curds, and natto, fermented soybeans, may not be staples in your kitchen. But maybe they should.

Soy isoflavones daidzein and genistein found in foods like tofu and natto were associated with improved sleep quality and duration in a study of 1,076 Japanese adults. Those who ate more soy foods on a daily basis slept better than those who ate the least.

Why? Isoflavones work like estrogen, which may help other chemicals in your brain regulate the sleep-wake cycle. Experts also suggest that the isoflavones may act as antioxidants to battle oxidative stress — a possible risk factor for poor sleep.

> Nine essential amino acids help keep your body healthy. Guess which food contains all nine? Soybeans. As you digest soy protein, those amino acids get picked up in your blood and put to good use throughout your body.

Not getting enough sleep has been shown to negatively impact cognitive functions like memory and attention. So next time you're looking for a snooze-friendly snack, grab a cup of isoflavone-rich soy milk before bedtime.

Count up your soy protein to cut down your cholesterol. Researchers reviewed the findings of 43 clinical trials involving 2,607 adults and found that soy protein reduced total cholesterol and low-density lipoprotein (LDL) cholesterol.

That's great news for your peace of mind, because too much cholesterol can block your arteries and deprive your brain of the oxygen-rich blood it needs to survive.

The median dose among study participants was 25 grams of soy protein a day. What does that amount look like? If you ate a soy burger with 10 grams of soy protein, drank a cup of soy milk containing 6 grams, and ate 1/4 cup of soy nuts at 12 grams, you would be on target.

BRIGHT IDEA

Delectable ways to dine with soy

Looking for ways to make your diet more nutritious and exciting? Then go beyond the traditional soy milk, soy yogurt, and soy nuts. Try roasted soybean flour called kinako. It adds a warm, nutty flavor to oatmeal, shakes, yogurt, or ice cream. These three other soy foods are worth a try, too

Edamame. To cook these young, green soybeans yourself, look for them fresh or frozen, in the pod or shelled. Just throw out the pod when you eat the beans since it's too tough to chew — much like shelling and eating a peanut. Try adding your cooked soybeans to soups, salads, eggs, pastas, burritos, or chili.

Too much work? Pick up ready-made edamame hummus, pasta, or power bowls at your grocery.

Miso. Change up your routine with miso mayonnaise or salad dressing. If you're ready to cook with miso, you have flavor choices. Red miso offers the strongest kick, yellow yields a milder taste, and white is mellow and sweet. Use any of them as a base for soup or broth. Whip miso into mashed potatoes or mix it up to marinate meats or mingle with veggies.

Tempeh. It may look like a lightly colored brick, but this fermented soybean cake is a nutrient powerhouse. Buy it whole or make your own from a starter culture you can pick up at the grocery. Marinate it, then bake, grill, or saute it until the edges are brown and crispy. Use it as a meat substitute. Or serve it sliced, crumbled, grated, or cubed in your favorite dishes.

St. John's wort

This healing herb gives your brain an edge

People have long relied on plants to help ward off sickness, infections, and other ailments. One in particular — known as St. John's wort — has been used as far back as the ancient Greeks. Now scientists are realizing that this herbal remedy could help battle depression and improve your memory.

Beat the blues with this natural treatment. Past studies wavered back and forth about how effective St. John's wort is at fighting depression. But a large analysis published in the journal *Neuro-psychiatric Disease and Treatment* claims this plant may be just as powerful as certain prescription drugs. And even better? It appears to be safer, too.

Scientists analyzed 27 studies that compared St. John's wort and selective serotonin reuptake inhibitors (SSRIs), the most commonly prescribed type of antidepressant. They found that the herb was just as effective as SSRIs in treating mild to moderate depression in adults. Moreover, the authors noted that the St. John's wort users experienced fewer side effects.

If you're already taking antidepressants, steer clear of St. John's wort. Mixing the two could cause too much serotonin to build up in your body, which can lead to dangerous side effects. This herb can also interact with other prescription medications, so talk to your doctor before taking it.

Want to give your memory a helping hand? Try a little St. John's wort. Can't remember why you walked into a room? Or where you stashed your car keys? This herbal remedy may prevent that from happening.

Recently, researchers tested St. John's wort against a placebo. Eighty-two adults were given either a 250-milligram (mg) dose of St. John's wort extract or a 500-mg dose. An hour later they took tests that measured their short-term memory and attention span. All the participants repeated the experiment after taking a placebo in a separate session.

Results of the study indicate that, among all the volunteers, only the low dose of St. John's wort had a positive effect on memory. The researchers think this herb helps boost the level of dopamine in your brain, which improves your short-term memory.

BRIGHT IDEA

3 surprising ways to use St. John's wort

Want to put a fresh spin on old treatments? Try these new takes on St. John's wort remedies.

St. John's wort tea. Sitting down with a good book and a cup of hot tea is a great way to take the edge off. And it gets even better when you add St. John's wort to the mix. Pour a cup of boiled water over 2 teaspoons of dried St. John's wort. Steep for about 10 minutes, strain, and serve. If you want, you can add a dash of honey or lemon to taste.

Try an herbal jello. Want to make taking your medicine a sweet experience? Next time you make jello, swap out some of the water with a cup of St. John's wort tea and then follow the instructions on the box. Serve it up whenever you're feeling blue.

Whip up your own essential oil. Some people swear by the healing powers of St. John's wort oil for bumps and bruises. If you can get your hands on fresh plants, it's easy to make your own.

Allow the flowers to dry for a day before placing them in a glass jar and covering in olive oil. Leave the jar in a warm place for four weeks to let the oil soak up the nutrients. Strain the flowers and store the filtered oil in a dark place. You'll have a great essential oil to rub on your skin. Test on a small patch of skin first, just in case it causes any irritation. And don't add this oil to your food or drinks.

Strength training

Join the resistance — hone your mind when you tone your body

Do you think strength training is a young man's game? Think again. Staying fit and strong is one of the best ways to protect your body and mind from the effects of old age.

Bulk up to win the battle against dementia. Strength training — or resistance training — actually breaks your body down. Lifting weights, doing pushups, or performing other exercises that use resistance creates tiny tears in your muscles. But when your body repairs the damage, these muscles grow bigger and stronger. New research shows that these workouts strengthen more than your body, though.

A recent study found that strength training protects the areas in your brain that are vulnerable to Alzheimer's disease. Researchers divided 74 seniors with mild cognitive impairment into different groups that participated in resistance training, brain training, a combo of both, or a control activity two to three times a week.

At the end of the study, experts found that people who did resistance exercises performed better on cognitive tests and showed improvements in the parts of their brains involved in creating and storing memories.

Want to give your memory a helping hand? Hit the gym. Fading memory doesn't have to be a part of getting older. Scientists think exercise can help you hold on to your memories. Plus it may help you fine-tune your focus and organizational skills, too.

A new paper examined the exercise habits and brainpower of 3,535 adults. Researchers asked people about how often they worked out and then put them through a series of tests measuring memory and executive function, which involves abilities like attention, planning, and problem-solving.

They found that people who worked out at least once a week had better scores on their cognitive tests compared to people who never exercised.

Beat the blues by lifting weights. Experts say nearly 6 million seniors suffer from late-life depression. But new research may have uncovered how a simple, effective, and cheap remedy — exercise — keeps the blues at bay.

In a small study, seniors completed three weekly exercise sessions for 12 weeks. They spent one day doing high-intensity interval training on an exercise bike, and the other two days were spent doing strength training workouts.

Researchers already know that exercise improves mood and symptoms of depression. And this study revealed a possible reason — working out could help turn on certain genes in your muscles that your body uses to make mood-boosting compounds.

Flex your muscles to fend off these 3 diseases

Getting stronger is one of the best ways to stay lively in your golden years. Just ask Willie Murphy. The 82-year-old bodybuilder made national headlines when she fought off a would-be burglar. But foiling robbers isn't the only reason you should keep up with strength training. Exercise may help you fend off high blood pressure, sarcopenia, and obesity, too.

Strength training could beat back HBP. High blood pressure (HBP) is one of the most common causes of strokes and has long been linked with the development of Alzheimer's disease. There's good news, though. New research suggests that a little bit of exercise may be able to bring your blood pressure down.

Researchers recruited 39 senior women. Some of them had HBP, while others were within the normal range. They asked these women to complete two weekly weight machine sessions made up of leg presses, extensions, and curls as well as chest presses and low rows for 10 weeks.

At the end of the study, researchers found that some women had significant drops in their blood pressure while others didn't. The training improved their strength, though.

So weight training may be a powerful way to protect yourself from HBP. But even if it doesn't lower your blood pressure, you'll still improve your quality of life and overall health.

Want to stop sarcopenia? Double down on your protection with exercise and protein. As you age, your body tends to lose muscle mass. This process — which is called sarcopenia — is linked with poor brainpower. Fortunately, you can slow it down with a few simple tweaks to your diet and lifestyle.

A recent analysis of 19 studies found that resistance training and protein supplements helped improve muscle mass and strength in seniors at high risk of sarcopenia. Make sure to pair your workout routine with a protein-rich diet.

Build muscle to melt away fat. Obesity can cause conditions like diabetes, high blood pressure, and heart disease. And all three are bad news for your brain. If you want to lose a few pounds, don't shy away from lifting weights. Research suggests that strength training is actually a better way to shed fat while maintaining muscle than cardio alone.

Researchers divided 249 overweight older adults into three groups. Some were asked to follow a weight loss diet, while others combined the diet with either strength training or aerobic exercise.

At the end of 18 months, the scientists tallied up the data and found that people in the strength and aerobic groups lost more fat than the group that just dieted.

> The muscular system isn't the only powerhouse in your body. Your brain generates between 12 to 25 watts of energy, enough to power an LED lightbulb.

But the strength group lost less lean muscle mass than the aerobic group — a better change in body composition.

Want to try it yourself? People in this study did four 45-minute resistance training sessions every week.

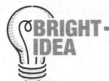

BRIGHT IDEA

Easy exercises for a complete home workout

Want to get a great workout without shelling out hundreds on exercise equipment? Resistance bands are exactly what you need. They're lightweight, versatile, and best of all — cheap. To get started, do three sets of these simple exercises.

Pallof press. Securely wrap one end of an exercise band around a doorknob or another stable, immovable object that's about chest high. With the other end of the band held close to your chest, walk backward until the band is stretched tight.

Turn to the right 90 degrees so the doorknob is by your side and push the band straight out. Hold this position for 15 seconds, then switch and do the same on your other side.

Band side step. Put a mini band or tie a long band around your thighs, just above your knees. Bend your legs slightly and place your feet hip-width apart.

Take a sideways step to your right until the band is stretched, then slowly slide your left leg until your feet are hip-width apart again. Repeat for 10 steps in one direction, then switch sides and work your left leg.

Band pull apart. Hold a resistance band straight out in front of you, with your hands shoulder-width apart.

Squeeze your shoulder blades together and slowly pull your arms apart until they are straight out and your body is in a "t" shape. Carefully return to the starting position and repeat 10 times.

Tai chi

Try this therapy for memory, sleep, and mood

Tai chi is a graceful form of gentle, low-impact exercise so simple anyone can do it. The series of stretching movements are performed slowly, allowing each position to flow into the next without interruption. This side effect-free therapy has been used for thousands of years to discipline the mind and body.

Some claim doing tai chi every day can work miracles to decrease your blood pressure, reduce inflammation, and temporarily ease chronic pain from arthritis. Not only that, this form of exercise has been found to reduce back, neck, and headache pain. Here's what else tai chi can do.

Meditative movements make memory stronger. The light physical exercises that are part of tai chi stimulate thinking ability and improve memory, possibly to heights you never dreamed possible. That's according to a study of 66 seniors with mild cognitive impairment.

Researchers gave the participants a memory test and then had an instructor teach half of them 10 tai chi moves over a three-week period. The participants then practiced at home over six months. By contrast, the rest of the volunteers received information on cognitive impairment and fall prevention. Researchers phoned the members of both groups weekly.

The result? At the end of the study, the tai chi group performed significantly better on memory tests than the control group. The researchers believe that their memories may have improved because they learned new skills, memorized movements, and switched tasks in order to perform the exercises.

Improve your sleep — no drugs needed. Even healthy seniors can have moderately severe sleep complaints. So researchers recruited 112 older adults and assigned a little more than half of them to 40-minute tai chi classes three times a week over four months. The remainder received general health education over a comparable amount of time.

After the study was over, the tai chi group experienced better sleep quality and longer sleep time. The control group's symptoms worsened. The results led researchers to suggest that these gentle exercises could achieve effects similar to sleep medicines, possibly before insomnia sets in.

Want to give tai chi a try? With practice, you can work through its fundamental moves in under 11 minutes.

Tai chi takes the edge off when you feel down. When you tackle chronic health problems with these basic moves, your mental health may improve, too. Studies suggest that regular tai chi practice can improve your mood and energy levels, cut back on your stress and anxiety, and help you with depression.

Researchers also put tai chi to the test against loneliness. They divided a group of socially isolated seniors into two groups. One attended hourlong tai chi classes twice a week for three months alongside their socially active neighbors. The other received occasional home visits by social workers.

Compared with the control group, the tai chi participants reported feeling significantly less lonely at the end of the study. Those feelings were still present three months later.

Has life got you feeling stressed out? Your brain may actually shrink when chronic stress upsets its delicate chemical and hormonal balance. You might also fall back on irrational ways of thinking and behaving. But experts say exercise, social connections, and learning help combat the effects of stress.

Leave the tumbling to the gymnasts — here's what everyone over 50 must know

Have you ever passed a park and noticed a group of seniors practicing simple, fluid movements and deep, rhythmic breathing? Most likely you've discovered a tai chi class. Don't stare — stop and join in. Those happy folks may be cutting their risk of falling and injuring themselves by as much as 50%.

That's according to a review of 10 studies on seniors and at-risk adults who practiced tai chi for an hour between one and three times a week over several months. Those results are encouraging given that more than a quarter of seniors over age 65 fall annually.

In fact, falls are serious business for several reasons. Even if they don't lead to dangerous and costly bone fractures, they can cause seniors to become fearful that another fall is just around the corner. Before you know it, you're changing up your routine and limiting what you do. That can lead to social isolation and cognitive decline.

So here's another reason why you'll want to take up tai chi. Researchers divided 368 seniors who had been treated for fall-related injuries into two groups — one that practiced tai chi and the other that focused on lower-extremity training to strengthen their hips, knees, and ankles.

Most of the participants met their tai chi group or physical therapist for 20 or more weekly, 60-minute sessions. They were reminded to practice daily, both during the study and after. At the end of six months, both groups responded well to the exercise by showing improved balance, muscle strength, and motor control.

But guess who saw the best results? The researchers found that the members of the tai chi group were significantly less likely to experience an injury-related fall than the lower-extremity training group — both at the end of the study and even a year later. Why was tai chi more effective? Experts suggest it improved the participants' hand-eye coordination, which helps you stay on your feet if you get a little wobbly.

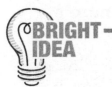

BRIGHT IDEA

Go with the flow and let tai chi classes get you moving

According to legend, a Chinese monk invented tai chi after witnessing a battle between a crane and a snake. Just as one animal swiftly attacked, the other smoothly evaded the blow. The fascinated monk eventually worked these and other animal movements into a low-intensity exercise routine that is now practiced around the world.

Experts say all you need is a little more than two hours of practice a week over six months to gain the brain benefits of tai chi. And its gentle, rhythmic movements can be adapted to suit many physical abilities. Some may find it necessary to use a chair as support, for example. Instructors recommend that you check with your doctor before starting a program so you can spot any challenges tai chi might pose.

Ready to get started? You can find free tai chi lessons online or buy an instructional program on DVD. But taking a class in person gives you the advantage of personalized attention.

Check out Supreme Chi Living, a website maintained by the American Tai Chi and Qigong Association, at *americantaichi.net*. Look for the class locator on their home page. Not finding what you want online? Call community centers, gyms, fitness sites, senior centers, and tai chi studios in your hometown to ask about their offerings.

When looking for a tai chi class, you want a program with a friendly environment that makes you feel comfortable. It should include warmup exercises, controlled breathing, slow arm and leg movements, and an emphasis on coordination and balance.

Technology

Small screen, big benefits: Stop your memory from short-circuiting

You may notice you spend more time watching a screen than your parents, or even you, did just 10 years ago. That's the trend right now for older Americans. On average they spend more than half of their seven hours of daily leisure time with a screen. Fortunately, you can use this tech to keep your brain active and alert.

Surf the web for an inflow of brain benefits. If you've been hesitant to purchase a cellphone or computer, now may be the time to buy in. Scientists followed over 13,000 people age 45 or older and found that owning these devices is associated with a lower risk of cognitive decline. And owners of both fared better than those with only one. The longer you have your gadget, the stronger the protection may be.

So what can you do on those devices to help your mind? Browsing the net is one option to help make your brain more resilient against mental aging. Using the internet gives you the opportunity to improve your health knowledge and reasoning skills or join social media for relationship benefits. You can also use email and cognitive training programs or games.

Computer use gives you a new memory card. Keeping your brain active by using a computer may offer benefits against age-related memory loss called mild cognitive impairment (MCI). This condition has milder symptoms than dementia. But even though people with MCI won't have their daily life significantly disrupted, they may find themselves losing their train of thought or have trouble remembering things.

You may be able to lower your risk of developing MCI as one study of adults age 70 and older has found. The seniors completed a questionnaire about how often they participated in mentally stimulating activities throughout their middle ages and older years. They also took thinking and memory tests throughout the study.

From these evaluations, the researchers determined using a computer is associated with a lower risk of developing thinking and memory problems. In fact, the chances were 37% lower for those who used a computer in both middle age and later life.

Stimulating leisure activities may make changes in your brain that help it deal with the threat of Alzheimer's disease. People who engage in mentally challenging hobbies may also have a healthy diet, an exercise routine, and good emotional health which also protect the mind.

3 tech tools that back your body and brain

Some gadgets help you stay more independent, active, and stress-free. Then there are tech tools that remind you to take your meds. Still others keep tabs on your blood pressure. Invest in technology that makes it easier to stay healthy and you'll help your brain perform at its peak.

Remote monitors help you age in place. Keeping active and independent around the house paves the way for better brain function. But sometimes staying in your home can be a challenge, especially if your children are worried about your well-being and want you to move or hire help. What can you do?

Remote monitoring systems may be a solution. Monitors range from sensors that only alert your family when you're up and about to cameras that let them drop in remotely to check on you.

Never miss a dose with medication reminders. Not sure if you took your medicine today? Sometimes keeping track of your pills seems harder than juggling a dozen balls. While you work on improving your memory skills with tips from this book, leave some of your worries to these memory savers.

- Phone call services can help you remember your meds. For a small monthly fee, you can set up daily calls to remind you it's time for a dose. Prices range from $4 to $30 monthly, and the more expensive options also monitor your health and safety.

- Smart pillboxes sound alarms and automatically dispense your pills when it's time for a dose. You'll pay about $20 and up for dispensers you fill and program yourself. The more complex devices have monthly subscription fees starting around $60. These are usually linked with services that call or text your loved ones if you miss a dose.

Wearable gadgets keep track of your vital signs. With a single payment of a few hundred dollars you can get a smart watch or wearable gadget that lets you keep an eye on your own vitals. Devices that once only gave you medical readings, like glucose monitors, are also getting high-tech makeovers. These upgrades sync with your phone. That makes it even easier for you to monitor your health and keep an eye on areas like blood sugar that impact your brain.

The prices depend on what device you go for, and some options are only available with a prescription. A few of the high-end products even send alerts to medical professionals if they detect potential health problems.

Trade TV mind melt for active alternatives. One study shows older adults who passively watched TV for 3 1/2 hours or more every day had greater verbal memory decline than those who watched less. Try swapping TV time for mentally stimulating activities like playing board or video games and reading books.

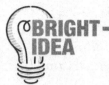

Keep your mind organized with these apps

Ever wish you had a personal assistant to keep track of your schedule for you? Your smartphone may be the perfect alternative. The myriad features might seem overwhelming at first, but these four apps come installed on your device. Delegate simple tasks to them, so you can stay focused on other priorities without missing a thing.

- Calendar. Quick! As soon as you leave the doctor's office mark your next appointment and set up a reminder. Use this tool to keep track of household events, too, like when your exterminator is coming. And you'll never forget to change the filter on the air conditioner if you keep all the dates in this one handy place.

- Alarm. Don't miss your appointments. Set your cellphone alarm so you'll be ready to go in plenty of time. Schedule an alarm for your medication times, too, so you won't miss another dose. Check for a "repeat" option so you don't have to continuously reset the alarm. It will automatically ring at the same time every day.

- Calculator. Have trouble keeping track of numbers in your head? Turn to your phone's calculator for help, and you'll always gets the right answer.

- Notes. A different password for every account sounds like a good safety precaution until you don't remember all of them. Save yourself a headache and store your passwords in your phone's notes app, protected by a single security code. You can also use it to record addresses, lists of errands, and important reminders.

Turmeric

3 ways this golden spice hones your mind

Turmeric is all the rage these days. You can find this simple spice in supplements, teas, and even juices at grocery stores across the country. And there's a good reason for that — research shows turmeric offers up serious brain-boosting benefits.

Pile on the turmeric to ward off Alzheimer's. Want to win the war against Alzheimer's disease (AD)? Call on a spice you may have in your pantry right now. Turmeric — the golden spice that gives curries their distinct yellow color — is prized for its antioxidant and anti-inflammatory powers. And experts think this spice may keep your mind in tiptop shape, too.

Research suggests curcumin — the main active ingredient in turmeric — prevents the formation and growth of beta-amyloid plaques found in the brains of people with AD. Even better? Scientists have found that it may be even more successful at stopping new plaques from forming in your brain than the nonsteroidal anti-inflammatory drugs ibuprofen and naproxen.

Spice up your memory with curcumin. Your memory may not work as well as it used to. But this spice may bring it back to fighting form.

A recent study in the *American Journal of Geriatric Psychiatry* found that curcumin supplements helped improve the memories in seniors with mild cognitive impairment. Forty older adults with this condition had their cognitive abilities assessed and then were asked to take either 90 milligrams (mg) of curcumin twice a day or a placebo.

At the end of the 18-month study, the researchers retested the seniors. They found that, compared with the control group, those taking curcumin had significant improvements in their ability to remember things and pay attention. The authors think curcumin helps reduce inflammation in the brain associated with memory problems.

Want to try it yourself? You'd have to eat 2 teaspoons of turmeric a day to get the same amount of curcumin. If you want to take a supplement instead, talk to your doctor to see if that could work for you.

Feeling blue? Improve your mood naturally. Don't let depression dog your golden years. Research from the *Journal of Affective Disorders* says turmeric may lift your spirits. In a small study, scientists asked people with severe depression to take either 500 mg of curcumin supplements twice a day or a placebo.

At the end of eight weeks, the researchers found that curcumin was a lot more effective than the placebo in improving symptoms of depression. They say this compound may help fight off the high levels of inflammation often found in people with severe depression.

Pile on the turmeric to tackle this triple threat

Wouldn't it be great if there were a single food you could eat to prevent cancer, fight off heart disease, and ease arthritis pain? Amazingly, there is — turmeric. This interesting spice does it all. It's packed with antioxidants that can help you stay in tiptop shape in your golden years.

Want to crush your risk of cancer? Enlist the help of curcumin. A recent analysis published in the journal *Nutrients* suggests that curcumin may be able to help fend off cancers all over your body.

Experts think inflammation can drive the development of cancer. That's because this condition causes your body to create chemical compounds that can kick-start the growth of cancerous cells. But curcumin helps block those compounds, so experts think it may help lower the risk of breast cancer, lung cancer, and other forms of this disease.

Researchers say more studies need to be done, so keep your eyes peeled for more information in the future.

Turmeric helps you stay ahead of heart disease. Ancient Greeks believed that the heart — not the brain — was the center of thought. While you know that's not true, the two organs are strongly linked. In fact, a growing body of evidence suggests that heart disease may increase your risk of dementia.

Of course, cardiovascular disease can also lead to fatal heart attacks and strokes. But turmeric may help prevent all that. Scientists polled over 44,300 people about the foods and spices they ate. Then, they tracked them for 11 years. Researchers found that the people who reported eating turmeric regularly were less likely to die from heart disease than those who didn't.

Banish joint pain with this natural remedy. Aching joints aren't an inevitable sign of aging. A key ingredient in turmeric can help keep arthritis at bay.

Scientists recruited 139 people with osteoarthritis (OA) in their knees and asked them to take either curcumin supplements or a prescription pain medication. At the end of the 28-day study, researchers found that the people who took the curcumin had similar levels of pain relief as those who took the drug.

The volunteers took 1,500 milligrams of curcumin every day. You'd need to eat roughly 1/3 cup of turmeric a day to get that through your diet, so talk to your doctor about supplements.

And protecting your joints is good for more than just your body. A recent meta-analysis shows an association between OA and a higher risk for dementia. Researchers say the link could be due to harmful molecules called cytokines that promote inflammation. Fortunately, curcumin helps block these compounds.

Ever hear someone say humans use only 10% of their brains? Turns out that's a myth. Scientists say you actually use all of your brain. Even sleeping takes up more than a tenth of your brainpower.

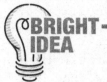

BRIGHT IDEA

This one-two punch can help you win the battle against dementia

Remember stirring cocoa powder into milk for an after-school treat? If you loved drinking chocolate milk, you might want to try this grown-up version. Golden milk, made by mixing turmeric and other spices into your drink, is a tasty treat that can help keep your brain healthy.

That's because turmeric is loaded with curcumin, and milk is packed with vitamin D. Here's how you can combine them to load all your protection into one super drink.

- Bring 1 cup of milk or nondairy milk to a simmer in a small saucepan. If you go with a nut milk, just make sure it has plenty of vitamin D.

- Whisk in 1/2 teaspoon of ground turmeric. You can add a bit more if you want a stronger flavor. Or if it tastes too intense, dial the turmeric back a bit.

- Stir in a few of your favorite spices. Try mixing in a dash of cinnamon, grated fresh ginger, whole cardamon pods, or even a pinch of black pepper. Want it sweet? Try adding a spoonful of honey.

- Strain out any solids and give it a final stir to combine. Serve warm or chill in the fridge.

Vaccinations

Vaccines: A shot in the arm for your brain health

Do you remember lining up with your elementary school classmates to receive an unexpected treat? A sugar cube, dipped in a pink polio vaccine, that tasted sweet to you — and provided sweet relief for parents who lived in fear of the debilitating disease that could put their child in braces, a wheelchair, or even an iron lung. A miracle medicine? Definitely. That vaccine cube, first used in the 1960s, helped eliminate polio from the United States by 1979.

Vaccines are just as important today as they were decades ago. But not only are they protecting you from illnesses like the flu and pneumonia, they're also tied to a lower risk of Alzheimer's disease (AD). How about that for some sweet relief?

Past exposure to these vaccines have made the headlines.

- A new study presented at the Alzheimer's Association International Conference suggests that getting at least one flu vaccination was associated with a 17% reduction in AD. More frequent flu vaccinations were linked to another 13% drop in AD.

- The same study shows vaccination against pneumonia between the ages of 65 and 75 reduced AD risk by up to 40% depending on the person's genetic makeup.

- A separate study of 3,865 seniors 65 and older showed that vaccines against diphtheria or tetanus, and against polio, were associated with 60% and 40% lower risk, respectively, of developing AD.

Researchers aren't sure what causes this positive side effect of vaccines, but they suggest that folks who keep up with their shots may maintain a healthier lifestyle in general.

"It may turn out to be as simple as if you're taking care of your health in this way — getting vaccinated — you're also taking care of yourself in other ways, and these things add up to lower risk of Alzheimer's and other dementias," says Maria C. Carrillo, Ph.D., Alzheimer's Association chief science officer.

Needle your way to your healthiest life with these 4 vaccines

Are you in your golden years? Then get ready to roll up your sleeves. It's time to get yourself vaccinated against four serious diseases that could really knock your socks off.

You may be surprised to learn that the illnesses these vaccines help prevent are tied to conditions like high blood sugar, infections, and blood clots — all of which could have an impact on your brain health.

Fend off the flu to keep your health in check. Getting the flu vaccine can cut your risk of getting the flu by up to 60%, which lowers your chances for life-threatening complications. And it helps you avoid those dreaded hospital stays.

This vaccine is especially important if you have diabetes. Even if you're managing the condition well, diabetes can make it harder for you to fight infections, which puts you more at risk for serious side effects. For example, some illnesses like the flu can cause your blood sugars to rise to dangerously high levels.

Pneumococcal vaccine shields against numerous conditions. This vaccine with the hard-to-pronounce name will protect you from several serious complications, including pneumonia, ear infections, sinus infections, meningitis, and other bacterial infections.

Most pneumococcal infections are mild, but some can cause long-term problems, like hearing loss or even brain damage.

Two vaccines are used against pneumococcal disease, Prevnar 13 and Pneumovax 23. The Centers for Disease Control and Prevention suggests adults 65 and older get both shots a year apart. Once you get these shots, though, you're good for life.

Single out perks for your heart and mind with the shingles shot. The culprit in shingles is the chickenpox virus, found in almost all adults who had the itchy disease as a child. The condition comes with a blistering rash that usually clears up in two to four weeks. And some people may experience nerve pain, referred to as PHN, that can continue for months. Shingles has also been found to raise the risk of stroke by 35% and the risk of heart attack by 59%.

But the shingles vaccine, recommended for adults over the age of 60, can spare you all that discomfort. Researchers are still studying how long the vaccine will be effective.

Tap into the many benefits of Tdap. Vaccines against tetanus, diphtheria, and pertussis are all wrapped up in this shot. The Tdap is actually the booster shot for the childhood DTaP. If you didn't get one as a teen or adult, get it now. This vaccine is especially important if you plan to spend time around a child younger than 12 months.

If you got a Tdap more than 10 years ago, experts say it's time for diphtheria and tetanus boosters. A Tdap vaccine can help you avoid some pretty serious complications including breathing difficulties, blood clots, or changes in blood pressure and heart rate.

> Since flu season normally starts in late October, early fall is the best time to get vaccinated. And if possible, get your shot in the morning between 9 a.m. and 11 a.m. One study showed that vaccines given at that time produced higher levels of antibodies than those given later in the day.

Valerian

The centuries-old herb that uproots uneasy moods

Valerian's lightly vanilla-scented flowers were used to make perfume hundreds of years ago, but it's the root system that counts when it comes to this plant's mighty medicinal powers. Here's how this ancient herb can lighten your mood.

Slough off stress with this root. Despite the pleasant fragrance of valerian's flowers, the roots are known for an unappealing scent. Fortunately, you don't have to eat the roots to gain their health benefits. Valerian root extract (VRE) is available in pills and capsules, and has been studied for its effect on people experiencing psychological stress.

In one study, participants were given either a 100-milligram VRE pill or a placebo three times a day over four weeks. Both the placebo and VRE groups showed improvements in their anxiety symptoms. But differences appeared when their brain waves were examined.

Researchers found that the people who took VRE had significant increases in their alpha wave activity. These brain signals reflect a relaxed state of mind. The VRE group also saw a decrease in theta wave activity. Some studies link these waves to negative thoughts and emotions.

The researchers say valerian may have caused a reduction in anxiety by helping the participants process their feelings.

Ease anxiety with this herbal supplement. You may have wondered if valerian is as effective as prescription medicines. One study set out to find just that. Researchers examined the effects of valerian on people with generalized anxiety disorder (GAD) — a condition that causes people to have unfounded, persistent worries that interfere with daily life.

The scientists compared their results with those of a control group that took a medication used to treat depression and anxiety.

After four weeks of treatment, both groups experienced a decrease in their anxiety symptoms. They also had lower levels of the primary stress hormone cortisol than at the start. Cortisol levels, which rise when your brain senses a threat, put your body on high alert. Too much of this hormone can cause you to feel anxious.

Some people have reported mild side effects like headaches and dizziness after taking valerian. That's why it's important to talk to your doctor before adding it to your routine.

This potent sleeping draught fights insomnia

Time travel back to ancient Greece and you'd see the physician Hippocrates prescribing valerian as a sleep aid. Hop forward to present day, and you'll find that modern science agrees with the father of Western medicine — this herb may well keep you from tossing and turning at night.

Most research suggests that valerian improves sleep quality — a measure of how long it takes you to fall asleep and how soundly you sleep through the night. It's great news for older adults as experts believe about half of seniors have sleeping troubles.

What's more, common menopause symptoms like hot flashes and night sweats — which can last well into your 60s and beyond — can make it even harder to get a good night's rest. So scientists studied the effects of valerian on 100 postmenopausal women with insomnia.

The volunteers were divided into two groups and received either 530 milligrams of concentrated valerian extract or a placebo twice a day. After four weeks, 30% of the women taking valerian extract had better sleep quality. That compares with just 4% of the group that took a placebo.

Not getting enough sleep has been shown to harm cognitive functions like memory and the ability to pay attention. So valerian may help your brain, too. Check with your doctor before trying it out because valerian can interact with prescription medications and increase the effects of other sleep aids.

Vegetarianism

Food for thought — 2 brain benefits of picking plants

Folks who choose not to eat meat and poultry call themselves vegetarians. While the first use of this name is a matter of linguistic debate starting in the 19th century, the principle of avoiding meat goes back to humanity's earliest days on the planet.

Vegetarians throughout the centuries have had a range of ethical, moral, religious, and health-based reasons for their food choices. Today science is backing them up with real data showing how a plant-based diet supports your emotional and mental health.

But being a vegetarian doesn't necessarily mean you only eat fruits, veggies, nuts, and whole grains. These vegetarian diets feature plant-based foods as the main dish but vary in what other foods they include.

Diet	Red meat and poultry	Fish and seafood	Dairy	Eggs
vegan	no	no	no	no
lacto-vegetarian	no	no	yes	no
ovo-vegetarian	no	no	no	yes
lacto-ovo vegetarian	no	no	yes	yes
pescovegetarian	no	yes	maybe	maybe
flexitarian	some	some	some	some

Eat more plants now to fend off cognitive decline later. Any of those types of vegetarian diets could serve your brain well over the long term according to one study out of Singapore.

For nearly 20 years, researchers tracked 16,948 people who were eating a healthy diet rich in plants. They found that those who stuck closest to their diets faced a lower risk of cognitive impairment later in life.

According to the experts, those eating habits may have lowered the risk for factors, like chronic diseases and inflammation, that are associated with mental decline. And fruits, vegetables, and whole grains also set the stage for a healthy gut microbiome, which supports brain health.

Have you heard the news? Plant eaters stress less than meat eaters. If anxiety gets the best of you, a Western diet could be the reason. Animal fats — along with refined grains and processed foods — are associated with higher levels of inflammation, which contributes to mood problems.

In a study, 620 healthy adults were assigned to one of three categories based on their usual diet — vegetarians, vegans, or omnivores who ate plants and animals. Those eating a plant-based diet reported better moods compared to those who were meat eaters. And vegans reported the lowest anxiety and stress scores. Experts say it may be because they favored fruits and veggies, had less alcohol and sweets, exercised more, and spent extra time outdoors.

Live longer and stronger when you cut back on meat

One diet for allover body benefits? Yes, please. Research points to plant-based diets as a way to decrease your risk of cognitive decline, in part by tackling conditions like these that put you at risk in the first place. Here's what they have found so far.

- Heart disease. An 18-year study of 70,696 adults concluded that people were less likely to die of heart disease when they replaced red and processed meat protein with plant protein.

- Stroke. Adults in Taiwan who ate a vegetarian diet had a lower risk of stroke. Researchers found these vegetarians also had lower blood pressure than nonvegetarians.

- Cholesterol. After switching to a partially vegetarian diet — called flexitarian — where 70% of the protein people ate was plant-based and 30% was animal-based, adults in Finland had lower cholesterol after only 12 weeks. Why? They were eating more fiber and fewer unhealthy dietary fats.

- Diabetes. Going vegetarian may prevent you from developing diabetes. And switching to a plant-based diet has helped people with diabetes lower or even eliminate their dosage of insulin medication.

- Weight. A review of 12 studies on plant-based diets and weight control found that participants achieved weight loss over about 18 weeks. How? They were eating foods that helped control their blood sugar, plus they were getting valuable antioxidants, minerals, and fiber.

BRIGHT IDEA

Nutrition know-how for vegetarians

Ready to switch to plant-based eating? You could start slowly by joining a campaign like Meatless Monday. Or maybe you'd rather be all-in from the beginning? No matter how you do it, put in a little planning time to make sure you're on top of your nutrition game.

- Pick protein to up your energy. Your vegetarian or vegan diet should substitute plant proteins that come from legumes, nuts, and seeds.

- Seek calcium for strong bones and more. Calcium is plentiful in dairy, but you may not get enough if you're following a vegan diet. Choose almonds, dark leafy greens like kale and spinach, figs, tofu, and oranges.

- Be on the lookout for B12. This nutrient helps keep anemia at bay. If you're going vegan, you can find B12 in fortified foods. Vegetarians should get plenty of it from milk, eggs, and cheese.

And watch your labels. Animal products may be hidden in seemingly innocent foods. Vegans should look for ingredients like gelatin, casein, whey, and even products used to soften bread like cysteine.

Video games

Play games to hone your mind

Video games aren't just for kids anymore. More than 50 million seniors love to play these electronic games known for their colorful graphics and fantastic sound effects — and for good reason. Research shows this pastime offers up some serious brain-boosting benefits.

Max out your memory stats in just two weeks. Ever hear someone say staring at a screen will rot your brain? Well they couldn't have been more wrong. In fact, it's scientifically proven that playing video games can actually improve your memory.

In a small study, researchers recruited a group of college students who didn't regularly play video games. Some were asked to play a three-dimensional (3D) game for half an hour a day for two weeks. Others were given a simple two-dimensional game, and the rest played neither.

At the end of the study, researchers discovered that the 3D group boosted their memory performance by a whopping 12%. However, the other two groups didn't see the same benefits.

The reason? Exploring the complex 3D world of video games may help improve function in the hippocampus, the region of your brain responsible for creating and storing memories.

Keep your brain young with this simple hobby. Video games can do more than give your memory a helping hand. A recent study published by Canadian researchers found that these games can actually help beef up your gray matter.

The scientists recruited 33 seniors and split them into three groups. Some were asked to play video games for half an hour a day, others took 30-minute piano lessons, and the last group wasn't given any tasks.

At the beginning and end of the six-month study, researchers tested the seniors' memories and scanned their brains in an MRI machine. They found that the video game players had increases in gray matter volume in the hippocampus, plus their short-term memory improved. The same wasn't true for the other two groups.

"3D video games engage the hippocampus into creating a cognitive map, or a mental representation, of the virtual environment that the brain is exploring," says study author Gregory West, a professor at the University of Montreal. "Several studies suggest stimulation of the hippocampus increases both functional activity and gray matter within this region."

Want to lift your spirits? Give video games a go. Video games are a great way to unwind after a long day. And a study shows this hobby may help you keep stress and anxiety at bay.

Experts polled a group of 140 seniors about their video game habits and put them through a series of tests designed to examine their social and emotional well-being. People who played video games reported higher levels of well-being. Those who didn't reported higher levels of depression and more negative emotions.

Level up your health with this surprising hack

Worried that taking up video games will turn you into a couch potato? A hybrid of video games and exercise — known as exergaming or active gaming — might just be the answer.

So how does it work? Some modern games come with balance boards, cameras, or other tech that allows you to control the game by moving your body. It combines the fun of playing your favorite games with benefits to your fitness and health. In fact, studies show these workouts can help fend off disease.

Dodge diabetes with help from active gaming. A recent study found that seniors with type 2 diabetes may lose verbal fluency and memory more quickly than those without the condition. One possible reason? High levels of circulating insulin may prevent the breakdown of beta-amyloid plaques that are linked with Alzheimer's disease. Fortunately, exergaming can help you manage diabetes.

A study published in the journal *BMC Endocrine Disorders* divided 176 seniors with diabetes into two groups. Some were asked to play a fitness-based video game every day for at least half an hour. Others were asked to stick with their regular lifestyle.

After 12 weeks, researchers checked back in with the seniors. They found that the group who played the video game had lower fasting blood sugar levels and reported a higher quality of life compared to the control group. And when the control group switched to the game, they had similar benefits.

Feeling frail? Exergaming can help you have fun and stay fit. Research suggests that adults who are frail — meaning they have fatigue, muscle weakness, and low levels of physical activity — are at a higher risk for cognitive decline. Exercise can help allay those concerns. But if you need a bit of extra motivation to work out, video games might have the answer.

In a small study, Taiwanese scientists asked seniors who showed symptoms of frailty to play an exercise-based video game or do traditional workouts three times a week.

At the end of the three-month study, they found that both groups improved muscle weakness, activity levels, and walking speed. However, only the exergamers improved their balance and energy levels.

> Video games are a great way to relax, but you don't want to go overboard. Spending too much time playing games could cause repetitive stress injuries to your hands and wrists. And staring at a screen without long breaks can cause eye strain. Set a limit on how long and how often you play.

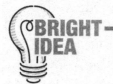

3 simple steps to choosing the perfect game

Ready to dip your toes into the world of video games? Use these top tips to get started.

Decide how you want to play. Some people love playing video games on dedicated consoles, like the Nintendo Wii or Sony PlayStation. However, these systems can costs hundreds of dollars, plus you still have to purchase games. You can look at used consoles, or ask around to see if anybody has one you can try before you buy.

You can get games for smartphones and computers, too. If you do buy a game to play on your laptop, make sure it's compatible before you splash the cash.

Follow your interests. Once you've found a way to play, you need to find the right game for you. Instead of going in blind, look for games that reflect your hobbies. Say you love bowling? Look at bowling games. If you need a bit more guidance, talk to an employee at a local video game store. They might help you pick beginner-friendly games, or even let you test them out before making a purchase.

Ask your friends and loved ones what they're playing. Reach out to your grandkids to see what they like. You could invite them over for a fun-filled Saturday afternoon of popcorn and video games.

Do they live far away? No problem. Some games let you play online, so you can use them to connect with people across the globe.

Vitamin B12

Ace your B levels for a stronger mind and body

Keeping your body's nerve and blood cells healthy, making DNA, and improving brain function all fall on vitamin B12's resume. Irritability, incontinence, dementia, and even numbness in your hands and feet could all be caused by a simple B12 deficiency that your doctor probably can't detect with a routine blood test. But replacing this important nutrient may help you feel much better in as little as two days.

Mend your mood with B12. Sleeplessness, moodiness, and depression could mean you aren't getting enough B12. Experts theorize that a lack of this vitamin contributes to high levels of the amino acid homocysteine, a condition associated with depression. But you can protect yourself by making sure you get sufficient amounts.

That's according to a long-term study that looked at the relationship between diet and depression in some 3,500 seniors. Researchers found that the participants who got more B12 and B6 from food and supplements were less likely to have depression than those who got less.

This vitamin helps you think more clearly. Feeling forgetful and confused? Try taking this one vitamin — B12 — to help with your memory problems. Researchers say it plays a key role in your brain's memory center, the hippocampus.

A study of older adults with mild memory problems suggests that even normal B12 levels may not be enough. The scientists found that seniors with B12 blood concentrations on the low side of the normal range performed worse on learning and memory tests than those whose levels were on the high end.

Don't let sarcopenia sap your strength. Losing your strength may be one of your greatest fears. After all, muscle weakness can lead to poor balance and falls and injuries. You may be able to fight off muscle weakness with B12, though.

To investigate this, researchers recruited 66 individuals age 65 and older with sarcopenia and matched them with the same number of older adults without the condition. The scientists found that the people with sarcopenia consumed significantly less B12 than those without muscle loss. In fact, 26% of the participants with sarcopenia were deficient in B12. That compares with only 11% of those without the condition.

It's not just your muscles at risk, either. This hardworking vitamin also helps prevent a blood disorder called megaloblastic anemia, which is why a deficiency in B12 may leave you feeling mentally and physically exhausted.

Got a deficiency? Here's the bitter truth about antacids

Those same antacids you rely on to relieve heartburn may have a surprising cost — a vitamin B12 deficiency. That's according to a huge Kaiser Permanente study that examined the connection between B12 levels and antacid use.

Researchers compared nearly 26,000 people who were deficient in B12 with 184,000 people who had enough of this vitamin. They found that those who used medication to reduce their stomach acid for at least two years were 65% more likely to have a vitamin B12 deficiency than those who didn't. That's not all. Among this group, those taking the highest daily doses were more likely to run short on this important nutrient.

The problem with antacids is simple — your stomach needs acid to properly absorb B12. So when you take medication that reduces acid production, your stomach's pH changes and makes B12 absorption more difficult. That's why the study participants' B12 levels rose when they stopped taking antacids.

Despite this potential drawback, you shouldn't skip prescribed medication. Instead check with your doctor about taking a lower dose. If you're experiencing symptoms of low B12 levels, you may also want to ask about screening for a deficiency in this vitamin.

Envision a way to keep your eyesight strong

Want to see your future more clearly? Keep your vision sharp by avoiding age-related macular degeneration (AMD) — one of the leading causes of vision loss in older adults. This eye condition affects the central part of the retina, called the macula.

Early symptoms of AMD include dark, blurry areas in the center of your vision. Late-stage AMD can leave you with an irreversible blind spot. Scientists have identified several contributing factors to AMD, including genetics, environment, and age.

Experts believe vitamin B12 may decrease the risk of AMD progression. One study followed up on seniors who had participated a decade earlier in a large Australian study on vision and common eye diseases. The researchers found that the seniors with low levels of vitamin B12 had a higher risk of both early- and late-stage AMD than those who got sufficient amounts. What's more, the participants who took a B12 supplement had a 47% lower risk of having AMD — at any stage — than those who didn't.

Supplements are an excellent choice for older adults who may have difficulty absorbing B12. That's because your body more easily absorbs B12 in this form than it does from food. So how does B12 help ward off AMD?

Vitamin B12 supplements offer numerous benefits, but you can still have too much of a good thing. Researchers have found an increased risk of hip fracture in older women who took high doses of B12 in combination with vitamin B6. That's why you should avoid exceeding recommended daily doses.

Researchers say the vitamin may improve how well the eye's blood vessels respond to outside stimulation — a process that's called vascular reactivity.

Here's another reason to get enough B12. Problems with the vascular, or circulatory, system can occur throughout the body. For instance, people with mild vascular disease that damages the retina are more likely to have problems with thinking and memory skills. Why? They may also have vascular disease in the brain.

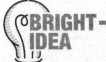

BRIGHT IDEA

12 top sources of B12

Your body can't make vitamin B12, so getting enough from food is one path to better health. This important nutrient is found naturally in a variety of animal products. Plant-based foods don't contain B12 unless they've been fortified. Carefully read the labels of fortified foods for their vitamin content — the value may vary by brand.

The daily recommended amount for adults is just 2.4 micrograms (mcg). So if you don't have dietary restrictions, the world is your oyster — or clam — if you're looking for B12.

Food	Amount	Vitamin B12 (mcg)
clams	3 ounces	84.1
beef liver	3 ounces	70.7
oysters, raw	3 ounces	13.8
chicken giblets	1 cup	13.7
sardines, canned	3.75 ounces	8.2
wild rainbow trout	3 ounces	5.4
sockeye salmon	3 ounces	4.8
tuna, canned	5 ounces	4.6
yogurt, low-fat	8 ounces	1.4
milk, low-fat	8 ounces	1.3
Swiss cheese	1 ounce	0.9
egg, large	one	0.6

Vitamin D

A medley of ways this D-lightful vitamin can save your brain as you age

Does sunshine on your shoulders make you happy? And maybe rainy days always get you down. Here's one reason why. When you're out in the sun, your skin is busily producing vitamin D, a doozie of a vitamin that can brighten your mood while it cuts your risk of cognitive decline and memory loss. And even if raindrops do keep falling on your head, you can still get the vitamin D you need through certain foods and supplements — sure to make you smile.

How much vitamin D do the experts say you need to stay healthy? They recommend that adults ages 19 to 70 should try to get 15 micrograms (mcg), or 600 international units (IU), every day. Over age 70? Go for slightly more — 20 mcg, or 800 IU.

A little extra sunshine brightens up your brain. Here's a scary stat. Seniors can see cognitive decline up to three times faster if they don't get enough vitamin D. In a study of nearly 400 folks with an average age of 75, researchers found that people with low vitamin D levels had higher rates of decline in episodic memory, the kind used to remember information about recent or past events. They also noticed a drop in executive function, the set of skills that help you focus and organize tasks.

Rev up your memory with the right amount of vitamin D. Researchers divided a group of 42 women, between the ages of 50 and 70, into three groups. Each group received a daily dose of 600, 2,000, or 4,000 IU of vitamin D3. At the end of one year, they found that memory and learning improved in the group that took 2,000 IU every day — that's about 50 mcg. The other groups didn't improve.

The women who took the higher amounts also showed a slower reaction time. That's why researchers warn high doses like these may have consequences such as raising the risk of falling and fractures. So before you load up on vitamin D supplements, talk to your doctor about the risks.

> Sitting by a sunny window on a winter's day seems like a great way to boost your vitamin D, right? Nope. Sunlight is made up of ultraviolet A and ultraviolet B (UVB). The UVB gets your vitamin D production going. But you can't get UVB through a window — in your house or in your car.

Don't let a lack of D bring you down. In a study of almost 4,000 older people, researchers found that a deficiency in vitamin D was associated with a noticeable increased risk of depression — 75% — over a four-year period.

The study authors think the results could be caused by the way vitamin D affects your brain. Structural and functional changes in the brain have been found in folks with late-life depression, but researchers think vitamin D may actually work to protect your brain from these changes. So let that sunshine in.

Beat back these common signs of aging with vitamin D

A dip in brain function may be the first thing that comes to mind when you think of aging. And getting enough vitamin D can help. But that's not all. This super nutrient mightily protects against three other common signs of aging. Weak bones? Check. Weak muscles? You got it. And it's necessary for your immune system to work properly.

Seems like that's a vitamin you'd want to take every day, right? You might be surprised to learn that possibly one quarter of Americans don't get enough of it. Just look at what they're missing.

Build up those bones. Make sure you're getting enough vitamin D in your diet to prevent osteomalacia, a softening of the bones. Osteomalacia happens because of a lack of vitamin D, a nutrient that helps your body absorb calcium — important for maintaining bone strength and hardness.

And research has shown that having adequate calcium and vitamin D is a great way to reduce your risk of fracture. It does this in part by helping you maintain your balance and lowering your chances of falling.

Multiply your muscle mass. And avoid sarcopenia, a condition that involves losing muscle mass and function. One of vitamin D's jobs is to bind to receptors on your muscles. This increases muscle size, which in turn improves strength and physical performance. But low vitamin D levels are related to loss of muscle mass and strength.

Seniors with a vitamin D deficiency — especially men — are at a higher risk of developing sarcopenia. Researchers think supplementing with vitamin D might prove to be an effective way to prevent and treat sarcopenia.

Upgrade your immune system. Your body's first line of defense against disease and infection — your immune system — relies on vitamin D to keep it healthy. In fact, vitamin D is so important for your immune function that low levels of D can cause you to be more susceptible to infections and conditions like tuberculosis, asthma, and chronic obstructive pulmonary disease (COPD). Even the common cold.

So now that you know vitamin D is critical for a sharp brain, strong bones and muscles, and a healthy immune system, what's for dinner tonight? Maybe some fish? Fatty fish, like tuna, mackerel, and salmon, are some of the best sources of D.

You can also find the nutrient in cheese and beef liver. And look for it fortified in foods such as orange juice, yogurt, and cereal.

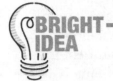

A tale of two Ds:
Which one do you choose?

You're shopping the supplement aisle in your local supermarket, looking for a bottle of vitamin D. You scan the well-stocked shelves. Vitamin A. A dozen different B vitamins. Vitamin C. Thank goodness all you need is D. Then you see it. Vitamin D2. Great. But wait. There's another bottle. Vitamin D3. Now you have to figure out the one that's right for you.

The difference between D3 and D2 in a nutshell? Vitamin D3 comes from animal products, like fish oil, butter, and egg yolk. And D3 is also made by your skin when you're exposed to sunlight. Vitamin D2, however, comes from fortified foods and plants, like fortified milk and mushrooms grown in ultraviolet light.

Researchers who compared the effects of vitamin D2 and vitamin D3 supplements on blood levels discovered that D3 raised blood concentrations of vitamin D more — and helped maintain those levels longer — than D2. And some experts claim vitamin D3 is a better form because it is naturally produced in your body.

When you're choosing a vitamin D supplement, look for the one that gives you the daily recommended allowance you need for your age group. Remember you need a little more as you get older because your body doesn't produce vitamin D as well. The Food and Drug Administration (FDA) now requires amounts to be listed in micrograms (mcg) instead of international units (IU).

Vitamin E

Brain bites: Foods that tell free radicals to take a hike

Got a favorite trail mix? Make your own vitamin E antioxidant super blend from sunflower seeds, peanuts, almonds, and dried cranberries and mangoes. It's a tasty snack to fight back against oxidative stress — an imbalance between unstable free radical molecules that can damage your cells and the antioxidants that fight them. This is especially important in your brain.

That's according to findings from the Rotterdam Study published in the *Archives of Neurology*. Over nearly 10 years researchers tracked levels of antioxidants like vitamin E in the diets of 5,395 people who were 55 and older. At the end of the study, those who ate foods with more vitamin E — a median of 18.5 milligrams a day — were less likely to develop dementia and Alzheimer's disease than those who ate the least.

"The brain is a site of high metabolic activity, which makes it vulnerable to oxidative damage, and slow accumulation of such damage over a lifetime may contribute to the development of dementia," the authors write. "In particular, when beta-amyloid (a hallmark of pathologic Alzheimer's disease) accumulates in the brain, an inflammatory response is likely evoked."

That response produces free radicals and can damage nerve cells in the brain. But the researchers conclude that vitamin E is a powerful fat-soluble antioxidant that may help block the development of dementia.

Newer studies have not found as strong a link between vitamin E and the risk of developing dementia. Though one study did find that vitamin E supplements slowed functional decline — problems with daily activities like shopping and preparing meals — in a group of people with mild to moderate Alzheimer's disease.

Researchers say it's too soon to recommend supplements for dementia just yet. But vitamin E-rich foods are a win-win — they're good for your body and may double as brain food, too.

Amp up antioxidants to protect your health in 2 ways

You need to fill up on the recommended 15 milligrams of vitamin E a day, and your body makes good use of it from there. This nutrient supports your immune system, helps widen blood vessels, and allows cells to carry out many important functions. Plus it can support your health in these ways.

Diabetes out of control? Get back in the driver's seat. A recent review of 12 studies looked at antioxidant levels in adults with type 2 diabetes. It concluded that supplementing with vitamin E — up to the safe upper limit of 1,100 mg a day — might help control diabetes complications related to blood vessel health.

How? Vitamin E fights damage to cells and blood vessel walls by breaking up free radical activity.

That's good for your brain, too. Blood vessel injury puts you at risk for vascular dementia. This type of dementia occurs from the brain damage caused by blocked blood flow to your brain.

Visualize stronger protection for your eyes. Poor vision can limit your ability to participate in activities that stimulate your brain. And what can hinder your vision? Low vitamin E levels.

But don't rely on supplements to protect your orbs. Only some studies have shown that vitamin E supplementation is linked to a

Vitamin E is an excellent antioxidant, but too much of it from supplements could increase your risk of bleeding or having a hemorrhagic stroke. Don't take more than 1,100 mg a day of either natural or synthetic vitamin E supplements unless directed by your doctor.

lower risk of age-related eye diseases like macular degeneration and cataracts.

However, experts at the American Optometric Association and the American Academy of Ophthalmology recommend including plenty of the antioxidant in your diet to support your eye health. Along with nuts and seeds, you'll find vitamin E in spinach, sweet potatoes, broccoli, and green beans.

BRIGHT IDEA

Now you're cooking — mix up your menu with nutrient-rich oils

Toss out your butter and make some room in your cabinet next to the olive oil. These oils packed with vitamin E are ripe for the picking — off the grocery shelf, that is. Check out what a single tablespoon has to offer your palate.

- Sample wheat germ oil for 20 milligrams (mg) of vitamin E. While not for cooking with heat, this oil adds strong nutty flavor to your morning oatmeal or yogurt. Some blend it into smoothies. Store it tightly sealed in a cool, dark spot.

- Got a hankering for nutty flavor? Try hazelnut oil in your coffee or drizzle it over crusty bread. A serving delivers a respectable 6.4 mg of vitamin E. Or grill your meat and saute your vegetables in it. This versatile oil performs at high heat and substitutes for butter.

- Turning up the heat with sunflower oil gets you 5.6 mg of vitamin E. Its light aroma won't get in the way of your food's flavors either. That makes it great for searing or sauteing. For an all-natural oil, look for the expeller-pressed kind, which uses a press to extract the oil rather than chemicals. It'll be more expensive, though.

- Almond oil offers 5.3 mg of vitamin E. For a flavor boost to cold dishes, use unrefined almond oil. Neutral-tasting refined almond oil is best when you add some temperature to your dish but has less of a nutritional punch. When you buy, pay attention to the label because some almond oils are sold specifically for skin care.

Volunteering

Mend your mind by helping others

You might find yourself with a lot of free time on your hands after retiring. If you're looking for another way to spend your days, why not try volunteer work? You'll improve your local community, give back to your neighbors, and — best of all — sharpen your mind.

Volunteering can beef up your memory. Who doesn't want to spend their golden years lounging on a beach? But after you hang up your briefcase, you need to make sure you don't go overboard with the rest and relaxation. Research suggests that staying engaged can help you keep your memory strong.

In a study published in *Alzheimer's & Dementia*, 111 seniors were divided into two groups. Some were enrolled in the Experience Corps, which meant they went into schools and helped mentor children, while others weren't.

At the beginning and end of the two-year study, scientists scanned the senior's brains to see if there were any changes. The control group showed signs of shrinkage in their brains. However, the volunteers actually had bigger brains than when the study started. And they also showed greater improvements on memory tests.

Study leader Michelle Carlson, Ph.D., points out that volunteering helped seniors work as part of a team, solve problems, and even get more physical activity. "We're not training them on one skill, like doing crossword puzzles," she says. "We're embedding complexity and novelty into their daily lives, something that tends to disappear once people retire. The same things that benefit us at 5, 10, 25, 35 — contact with others, meaningful work — are certain to benefit us as we age."

Soothe your mood when you help others. Giving back to others can give you a sense of meaning and purpose, which goes a long way toward lifting your spirits. In fact, British researchers published a study that revealed people who volunteer are often happier than people who don't.

They collected data from more than 5,000 households over the course of 12 years. People answered questions about how often they volunteered and how they rated their own mental health, including happiness, distress, and well-being.

The study revealed that people who donated their time tended to report better scores on their mental health assessments compared to people who never volunteered. And the more often they did volunteer work, the higher the scores tended to be.

Give and gain: Lend a hand for these life-changing benefits

Volunteer work is a great way to stay active and build social bonds as you age. And that's great news for your body and your brain.

Pay it forward to ditch disabilities. Not getting enough exercise can dramatically increase your chances of developing Alzheimer's disease. But as you age, you might find it harder to move around. Fortunately, research suggests that spending time volunteering is linked with better mobility in your golden years.

In the large-scale study, scientists looked at survey results from more than 13,000 adults over 14 years. The data included information about how often these people donated their time or worked, and the status of health and functional abilities — like climbing a flight of stairs and kneeling.

When they tallied up all the data, researchers discovered that people who worked or volunteered for up to 100 hours a year were less likely to develop chronic diseases or disabilities than those who didn't do either.

Feeling alone? Make new friends while helping your neighbors.
"Becoming a widow is one of the most difficult transitions that people face later in life," says Ben Lennox Kail, Ph.D., assistant professor of sociology at Georgia State University.

The stress and loneliness that come in the wake of such loss is linked with depression and an increased risk of dementia. Recent research suggests that volunteering may help you create social bonds and feel less lonely.

In the study, Kail and a team of researchers examined data on 5,882 adults who were at least 51 or older. Participants had reported how much they volunteered and how lonely they felt.

The paper revealed that people who had recently lost their spouse felt less lonely if they volunteered at least two hours a week. In fact, the authors of the paper noted that the difference in loneliness between volunteers who became widowed and volunteers who were still married was almost nonexistent.

> Donating your time in this day and age doesn't have to be done in person. Virtual volunteering opportunities let you help others from your phone, laptop, or tablet. Check out websites like *volunteermatch.org* and *allforgood.org* to find ways you can help.

Go back to work to dodge dementia

Many retirees say they would think about returning to work if conditions were right. Many others already have. In fact, one study found that 4 in 10 currently employed workers 65 and older had previously retired.

Why go back to work? It's not necessarily for the money. Some retirees miss the challenges, the accomplishments, and the connections they felt with former co-workers. Plus working longer may help keep your brain healthy.

In a recent study, Swedish researchers examined more than 63,500 seniors. And they found that a later-than-average retirement age was associated with a lower risk of dementia.

You can jump-start a part-time job search by contacting a former employer, searching the 50+ job boards, and checking your town's website for listings.

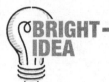

4 ways to get involved in your local community

Want to start volunteering but don't know where to sign up? Use this handy list to find opportunities near you.

Get involved with local students and youth programs. You can stay busy and help bridge the generation gap by volunteering your time and knowledge to students in high school. Nonprofits like Big Brothers Big Sisters of America also seek older adults with life experience.

"It's extremely gratifying," says Art Koff, who's been volunteering at *ICouldBe.org* for more than 15 years as an online mentor to inner-city students around the country. "I'd really urge any retiree who is computer literate to do it."

Feed your neighbors. Homebound seniors often have trouble buying and preparing healthy meals. So why not help out by signing up to deliver food with Meals on Wheels? Go online to *mealsonwheelsamerica.org/americaletsdolunch* to find an organization near you. Or check out *feedingamerica.org/take-action/volunteer* for opportunities at your local food pantry.

Venture into the great outdoors. The National Park Service gives volunteers the opportunity to work in some of the most beautiful places in America. And as an added bonus, volunteers get meals, stipends, and — if you work enough hours — a free park pass.

Go online to *nps.gov/getinvolved/volunteer.htm* to find out more. No national park near you? Reach out to local parks or wildlife centers to see if they need volunteers.

Don't forget about your public library. Libraries often offer a lot more than just books. Many run educational programs and they need people to help out. Ask if there are any ways you can donate your time.

Walking

Fancy footwork: 3 ways walking keeps you on your toes

"The Incredible Shrinking Brain" sounds like a frightfully bad horror film, doesn't it? Something about an alien invasion or with a psychotic creature in the credits. But hold on to your popcorn. This phenomenon is more of a documentary than fluff fiction.

Brain shrinkage is, in fact, a real thing, defined by the National Institutes of Health (NIH) as a loss of brain tissue including specialized nerve cells and the oh-so-important connections between them. This means if you suffer from cerebral atrophy — the technical term for brain shrinkage — your memory, ability to learn, and higher functions like planning and organizing could be damaged.

So what actually causes your brain to shrink? Could be damage from a stroke or head injury, an illness like multiple sclerosis, or even inflammation caused by an infection. But brains also shrink simply because they're getting older. It begins in your 30s and 40s, with different areas of your brain dwindling faster than others and certain factors worsening the problem — like stress, alcohol abuse, and high blood pressure.

Rewrite the ending of this motion picture reject with a simple activity you do every day. If you want to not only preserve your gray matter, but mend a host of other problems, experts say to put on your walking shoes.

Think better on your feet. Here are your choices — sit on the couch and have a smaller brain or take a walk and thwart Alzheimer's disease.

In research related to the landmark Framingham Heart Study, more than 1,000 people without dementia or heart disease took a treadmill test and had their heart rate and blood pressure measured. Twenty years later, they underwent a similar test, but this time also had MRI scans of their brains.

"We found a direct correlation in our study between poor fitness and brain volume decades later, which indicates accelerated brain aging," says Nicole Spartano, Ph.D., of Boston University School of Medicine.

If that's not convincing, consider the results of research recently published in the medical journal of the American Academy of Neurology. People who participated in aerobic activities like walking tested on thinking skills as if they were about 10 years younger at age 40 and about 20 years younger at age 60. Who wouldn't take a little ramble to turn back the clock like this?

"As people age, there can be a decline in thinking skills, however our study shows that getting regular exercise may help slow or even prevent such decline," says study author Yaakov Stern, Ph.D., of Columbia University in New York. "We found that all participants who exercised not only showed improvements in executive function but also increased the thickness in an area of the outer layer of their brain."

Step away from your energy crisis. It's raining. It's too hot out. Or, man, it's cold. All not-so-perfect excuses to forgo your daily walk. Don't let "Old Man Weather" beat you when you're feeling beat. Head for the stairs. Whether you're at home, in an office building, or somewhere in between, taking the stairs can punch up your energy level better than a jolt of caffeine.

A small study of sleep-deprived college women found they were more energized after resting for 20 minutes then climbing stairs for 10 minutes compared to either taking a caffeine pill then resting or simply taking a placebo capsule.

Walking barefoot can mean freedom from poorly fitting shoes that rub your heels and pinch your toes. Some even say your feet and ankles become stronger when they don't rely on shoes for support. But building your muscles and toughening your soles will take time. In addition, going shoeless leaves you vulnerable to injuries and infections. Reconsider especially if you have diabetes.

When you need a shot of energy or motivation, Patrick J. O'Connor, University of Georgia professor of kinesiology, says, "You may not have time to go for a swim, but you might have 10 minutes to walk up and down the stairs." And that's just enough time to fight fatigue, helping your brain stay focused and on task.

Don't lose your snooze. "Now I lay me down to sleep." Ahh, the classic bedtime prayer sure to bring on soothing rest and sweet dreams. But if your nightly routine continues with, "But I lay here counting sheep," perhaps you need to sashay your way into the land of Nod.

About 1 in 3 adults have trouble falling or staying asleep. If only they knew a night of quiet slumber was but a 10-minute walk away. For people who are normally inactive, that's all it might take to improve the likelihood of a good night's sleep.

Not getting enough sleep can lead to mood changes and anxiety, which in turn contribute to problems with memory. Experts say light exercise, like walking, is better than no activity and should be at the top of your list for healthy sleep habits.

Nature Rx: Walk green or blue to beat the blues

Start walking and you'll be healthier. Period. But combine your walk with a nature experience — in the forest or along a lake or river — and the mental health benefits simply explode.

Termed walking green or walking blue, these jaunts involve nothing more than trading the traffic for the trees, the sidewalk for the sand. There's no running involved and no cellphones allowed. You just walk and hopefully commune with nature.

In studies, blue and green walkers have reported improvements in their anxiety levels, mood, and energy, compared to when they walked in the city or along a busy street.

Step out today for a healthier heart

You began when you were just a year old, and you haven't stopped since. If you're like most Americans, you walk approximately 5,000 steps a day, or about 2 1/2 miles. That means by the time you hit 50, you've just about walked around the Earth's equator twice. No wonder you're pooped. But you're also healthier for all that walking. By simply continuing to put one foot in front of the other, you've engaged in an aerobic activity that strengthens your bones and muscles, burns calories, and slims your waistline.

But wait, there's more. Walking is a surefire winner when it comes to heart health.

BP TLC — take a walk in the fast lane. So just how borrrring is it to walk the same pace day after day after day? Well if you'd like to give your arteries a little extra love, it's time to liven that stroll up with something called interval walking. This means during your workout you alternate between periods of fast and normal paced walking.

The fast interval should be somewhat hard, defined as moderately to vigorously intense. Your heart rate is up, you're breathing deeply, and you probably can't talk while you're walking. Do this for three minutes then switch to three minutes at a more normal pace. Don't dillydally now — after all you're out for some exercise — but step to a more comfortable pace for this period.

Build your excursion around at least five sets of these six-minute combos and, presto, you've just packed in a 30-minute workout proven to do your arteries a world of good. Since stiff artery walls can cause high blood pressure (BP) — a leading cause of strokes — you've also just protected your brain from catastrophic damage.

Slow and steady wins this race. You don't have to be a marathon runner to reap exercise benefits. Over the course of six years, researchers kept up with 33,060 runners in the National Runners' Health Study and 15,945 walkers in the National Walkers' Health Study. And who do you suppose fared better when it came to heart health?

- The risk for high cholesterol was reduced more than 4% by running, but a whopping 7% by walking.

- The risk for heart disease was lowered 4.5% for the runners, but a little more than twice that for the walkers.

BRIGHT IDEA

Must-know tips to saunter safely

First get your doctor's approval to start a walking regimen, then follow these recommendations to keep your ramblings risk-free.

- At night, wear light, bright clothing with reflective material and carry a flashlight.

- Face oncoming traffic if you must walk in the road.

- Walk with a friend.

- Carry a cellphone.

- Invest in properly fitting shoes designed for walking.

- Choose a route free from debris, uneven surfaces, and other tripping hazards.

- If listening to music or an audiobook, always keep one ear free to hear traffic, sirens, and other noises.

Water

Check your fluids — top off your mind for better memory and mood

Here's an interesting fact about your amazing brain. Turns out 73% of it is made of plain old water. So if you get dehydrated by more than 2%, you can suffer from a loss in attention and other cognitive skills.

But staying hydrated is as simple as drinking eight glasses of water a day, right? Maybe. Experts say you might need anywhere from 8 to 15 cups of fluids daily — from water, other beverages, and food.

Unfortunately, as you get older your total body water decreases, which makes it easier for you to become dehydrated — sometimes before you even realize it.

Drinking water can go a long way to improving your memory. So why is it harder to pay attention to details when you're thirsty? Dehydration causes your body to work overtime to conserve water, borrowing fluid from cells to maintain other functions like blood flow. As a result, some cells may shrink and stop working properly.

Even mild dehydration affected performance on cognitive tests in two small studies. Compared to well-hydrated seniors, those who were dehydrated had worse scores on memory tasks.

Hydrate your way to happiness. If you're angry because you're hungry, folks call it "hangry." But did you know thirst is often mistaken for hunger? And the key to feeling better when you're dehydrated — obviously — is to drink more water.

Researchers asked 22 women who regularly drank a high volume of water — between 8 and 17 cups a day — to restrict themselves to only 4 cups daily for three days. Meanwhile, they asked participants who usually drank less than 5 cups of water a day to double their intake to about 10 cups daily for the same time period. The result?

The participants who drank the most water reported feeling better — more awake, less tired, and less confused. But those drinking the least water reported lower positive emotions and feeling less calm and content. Researchers say women may be especially sensitive to mild dehydration.

2 reasons to raise another glass of this life-giving liquid

Every living thing on the planet needs water to survive — and to thrive. Unfortunately, some researchers estimate that more than 95% of seniors in the U.S. don't drink enough water to be properly hydrated. And that can have dire consequences.

Drink more water to lose weight. Here's a shocker — being underhydrated is linked to obesity, according to one study. And obesity is tied to a higher risk of dementia. So how can H2O help your waistline?

In a study, researchers asked 50 overweight women to drink 2 extra cups of water 30 minutes before breakfast, lunch, and dinner for eight weeks — that was in addition to their normal amount. By the end of the study, they had lost weight and body fat. Their body mass index (BMI) and appetite had also decreased.

Stay hydrated to stand up to stroke. Studies have shown that hospitalized stroke patients were significantly more likely to have worse outcomes if they were dehydrated.

The journal of the Alzheimer's Association reports that, during the course of hospitalization or surgery, as many as 50% of older people experience delirium — a condition that affects attention and thinking and is associated with dementia. One of the risk factors for delirium is dehydration, so make sure you stay well hydrated.

"It's not clear why proper hydration at the time of stroke is linked to better stroke outcomes," says Dr. Mona Bahouth, stroke fellow at Johns Hopkins Hospital and lead researcher of one of those studies. "It's possible that dehydration causes blood to be thicker causing it to flow less easily to the brain through the narrowed or blocked blood vessels. The beauty here lies in the simplicity of this potential treatment. Rehydration is cheap and can be given to people even in the most remote locations."

The toxic truth behind sugar-sweetened beverages

There's no sugar-coating it. Americans eat too much sugar. Experts say the average person indulges in about 130 to 150 pounds of the sweet stuff each year. That's like chugging 7 to 8 cups of Hershey's Chocolate Syrup every week. And the leading source of added sugar in the American diet? Sugar-sweetened drinks.

It's not just kids and teens, either. According to the Centers for Disease Control and Prevention (CDC), on any given day, 5 out of every 10 adults drink a sugar-sweetened beverage. And it's ruining your health.

Refined sugars are toxic to your brain. They affect your thinking skills, memory, mood, and stress levels. Some scientists believe sugars, like fructose, actually block your brain cells from communicating properly. Others say it's all about the inflammation fructose causes and the damage it does to your blood vessels. The bottom line is this — if you load up on high-carb, high-calorie foods, you're raising your risk of brain shrinkage, dementia, and Alzheimer's disease.

Not so long ago, you only worried about sugar rotting your teeth. Now you have much bigger (and scarier) concerns — its link to a host of skyrocketing illnesses.

- **Worse than salt for your heart?** An article in a recent issue of the *American Journal of Cardiology* claims sugar may impact your blood pressure more than sodium. They say that sugar triggers your brain to speed up your heart rate and increase your blood pressure.

- **Sodas can make you fat.** According to a study out of the University of Southern California School of Medicine, foods containing added fructose, like sodas, can actually make you feel hungrier.

- **From wacky blood sugar to full-blown diabetes.** Fructose, specifically high fructose corn syrup (HFCS), is a big hidden sugar, added to thousands of processed foods, including cereals, baked goods, and sodas. Experts now think added fructose is more dangerous to the delicate insulin-glucose balance in your body than any other carbohydrate.

- **Who wants to look and feel older?** There's a new, alarming link between drinking sugar-sweetened sodas and life-threatening damage to the very structure of your cells. A study of more than 5,000 people found those who regularly indulged in sugary sodas damaged their DNA as much as if they smoked. Drinking a single 20-ounce soda daily made their bodies almost five years older. This damage also means you're more likely to develop any number of chronic diseases, including heart disease, diabetes, and some types of cancer.

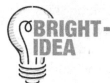

BRIGHT IDEA

With this healthy twist, soda can be yours again

What do you call your carbonated beverage — soda, pop, soft drink? Many doctors call them bad for you. There must be a healthier option, right? Here's how to make your own.

- Get your fizz from seltzer water. Don't confuse it for club soda or tonic water, which have added ingredients.

- Choose your sweet. Puree your favorite fruit with water, and strain. For extra sweetness, make a syrup from equal parts honey and water heated until combined. Blend the juice with syrup to taste.

- Pour your flavor over ice and top with seltzer. Store in the fridge.

Weight loss

2 brain-saving reasons to slim and trim down

Every year, losing weight ranks as the most common New Year's resolution. Then, 365 days older and a few pounds heavier, people make the same resolution again. While that extra weight puts you at extra risk for health problems, including diabetes, heart disease, high blood pressure, and certain forms of cancer, it can also impact your brain health. So ring in the next new year the right way — with a smart, healthy approach to weight control.

Watch your waistline to keep your memory sharp. Scientists discovered that having a high body mass index (BMI) — a measurement that uses your height and weight to determine body fat — may put you at risk for developing memory problems.

Chronic inflammation is your body's response to unhealthy lifestyles — living with too much stress, too little exercise, or too much fluff around your middle, for example. And now experts know that people with certain markers of inflammation at middle age are more likely to experience brain shrinkage and poor memory as they get older.

How do you help your brain bounce back? Drop a few pounds. One study showed that memory performance significantly improved after overweight women lost an average of 17 pounds.

Prevent bad-mood belly fat. You may feel unhappy when you're carrying a few extra pounds around the middle, but it's not all about dissatisfaction with your body. Belly fat also changes your body chemistry to make depression more likely. And the problem could go both ways, since some antidepressant drugs can make you gain weight.

No-nonsense numbers: BMI delivers healthy guidelines

Your body mass index (BMI) helps to determine if you are at a healthy weight for your height. To learn your BMI, find your height and weight on the following chart.

Body Mass Index (BMI)										
Light shading = overweight / Dark shading = obese										
Weight	100	110	120	130	140	150	160	170	180	190	200
Height										
5'0"	20	21	23	25	27	29	31	33	35	37	39
5'1"	19	21	23	25	26	28	30	32	34	36	38
5'2"	18	20	22	24	26	27	29	31	33	35	37
5'3"	18	19	21	23	25	27	28	30	32	34	35
5'4"	17	19	21	22	24	26	27	29	31	33	34
5'5"	17	18	20	22	23	25	27	28	30	32	33
5'6"	16	18	19	21	23	24	26	27	29	31	32
5'7"	16	17	19	20	22	23	25	27	28	30	31
5'8"	15	17	18	20	21	23	24	26	27	29	30
5'9"	15	16	18	19	21	22	24	25	27	28	30
5'10"	14	16	17	19	20	22	23	24	26	27	29
5'11"	14	15	17	18	20	21	22	24	25	26	28
6'0"	14	15	16	18	19	20	22	23	24	26	27
6'1"	13	15	16	17	18	20	21	22	24	25	26
6'2"	13	14	15	17	18	19	21	22	23	24	26
6'3"	12	14	15	16	17	19	20	21	22	24	25

If your BMI isn't in the healthy range, notice which weight numbers are healthy for your height. But remember, just as two heads are better than one, BMI is more valuable when it doesn't work alone. Here's why.

- BMI can give false readings for people with very high amounts of muscle like athletes or weightlifters, or unusually low amounts of muscle that may appear in some overweight women over age 50.

- BMI may be less accurate for people age 65 and up.

- BMI doesn't tell how much dangerous visceral fat you have. Visceral fat increases your risk of disease.

To help solve some of these problems, experts recommend you combine BMI with measuring your waist. This helps you estimate overall fat, as well as visceral fat.

Fight deadly duo with smart weight loss

Small weight loss steps lead to big life changes. Believe this and you can turn your health around. Ready to give it a try? Start making modest lifestyle adjustments that result in steady weight loss, and you'll triumph over two brain-sabotaging health conditions.

Don't let high blood pressure do a number on your noggin.
Dementia and mild cognitive impairment (MCI) — a condition marked by memory loss that may eventually lead to Alzheimer's disease — can be caused by blocked blood flow to the brain. Just the sort of thing that happens when high blood pressure damages your arteries.

New findings from the SPRINT MIND study, reported at a recent Alzheimer's Association International Conference, suggest that keeping your blood pressure under control may lower your risk of developing MCI and dementia.

"This is something doctors and the majority of their patients with elevated blood pressure should be doing now to keep their hearts — and brains — healthier," said Dr. Jeff D. Williamson, chief and professor of Geriatrics and Gerontology at Wake Forest School of Medicine. "These new results for maintaining cognitive health provide another strong rationale for starting and maintaining healthy lifestyle changes in midlife."

So protect your brain and your heart by getting your systolic blood pressure below 120 mmHg. And the No. 1 thing you can do to achieve this is to lose weight. Even dropping just a few pounds can substantially reduce your risk of developing high blood pressure.

One study found that women who had a BMI of 31 or higher were more than six times as likely to develop high blood pressure as women with BMIs less than 20. Even women with a BMI of 20 to 20.9 had a significantly higher risk. In fact, a one-point increase in BMI was associated with a 12% increase in risk for high blood pressure.

In the study, women who lost between 2 and 4 1/2 pounds lowered their risk by 15%, and women who lost more than 4 1/2 pounds lowered their risk by 26%.

An exercise routine to lose weight and lower your BP doesn't have to be excessive — aim for half an hour a day. Start by simply getting out of your chair. You can lower your systolic blood pressure just by breaking up long periods of sitting with a little exercise — take a walk or go for a swim. Working out in warm water dilates your blood vessels and improves blood flow, making it a great way to get fit and relax.

Fight diabetes one pound at a time. People with diabetes must keep an eye on a very special number. Your hemoglobin A1c, also known as HbA1c, tells your average blood sugar level over the past two to three months by showing the amount of glucose attached to the molecules in your red blood cells. The thicker the coat of sugar, the higher your HbA1c.

Having high blood sugar over time can harm the blood vessels that carry important nutrients to your brain, like oxygen and glucose. Getting your HbA1c below 6.5% — and keeping it there — can guard your memory, preserve your concentrating and learning abilities, and protect you from dementia.

A cycle of two weeks on your diet and two weeks off could have you dropping more pounds than if you dieted continuously. This is according to a study published in the *International Journal for Obesity*, which reported an intermittent diet group lost more weight than those dieting continuously, and gained less back after the trial was over.

So there's bad news and good news. Being overweight is the No. 1 risk factor for type 2 diabetes. And the heavier you are, the greater your risk. Is that enough to get you off the couch? Just consider the rewards.

If you have prediabetes and commit to boosting your physical activity just a little — say a 30-minute brisk walk five days a week — and dropping at least a few pounds, you could cut your risk for full-blown diabetes in half.

If you already have diabetes, simple lifestyle changes to lose weight could work wonders.

- Remember, glucose is energy. So when you're active, your body naturally uses it up. That means less glucose in your bloodstream triggering insulin production and wreaking other kinds of havoc.

- Dropping pounds by improving your diet and becoming more active could lower your blood pressure, cholesterol, and your risk of a devastating heart attack within the next five years.

Table talk: 5 unbelievably easy ideas to fast-track weight loss

Every meal is an opportunity to inch your way closer to your weight loss goals. Don't waste it.

- Measure your portions. The actual amounts of food you eat are often different from — and larger than — standard serving sizes.

- Slow down. It takes about 20 minutes for your brain to get the message your hunger is satisfied. Put your fork down between bites. Give your body time to get in sync.

- Stand up partway through your meal to see how you feel. Comfortably full? You've eaten enough. Feeling bloated? You've gone overboard. Learn your body's fullness signals.

- Focus on your food — not your screens. Turn off the TV and mute your cellphone.

- Don't skip meals, especially breakfast. Keeping to a regular schedule is the best way to ensure you won't get or stay hungry.

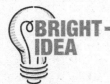

Winning after losing: Keep the weight off with proven tips

Don't want to regain the weight you worked so hard to shed? Then follow the lead of the "successful losers" enrolled in the National Weight Control Registry, an organization that tracks the habits of people who've dropped at least 30 pounds and kept it off.

"One of the key things for weight gain prevention is a regular pattern of physical activity," says Graham Thomas, Ph.D., an associate professor of psychiatry and human behavior at the Medical School of Brown University and a co-investigator at the Registry. "Our members, on average, do about an hour a day of brisk walking."

Thomas says exercise works double duty in helping you maintain a healthy weight. It burns calories and prevents some of the metabolic slowdown that accompanies aging and weight loss.

Of course, Thomas advises, it's important to eat a healthy, low-calorie diet. You should also keep track of what you eat and weigh yourself at least once a week.

"It gives you an opportunity to catch weight gain early before it becomes a major problem that's harder to reverse."

Any other secrets to successful weight maintenance? Most people on the Registry have breakfast, Thomas says, which likely helps them control hunger and avoid excessive eating later in the day.

They also tend to watch less TV than the average American. "It appears to be one way in which they have time to be physically active," Thomas says, adding that TV time also often leads to snacking.

Yoga

Put your body in motion to mind your mental health

How would you feel about a baby goat perching on your back while you struck a yoga pose? Many fans of goat yoga find it hilarious. So even if they don't get much of a workout, they walk away in a good mood.

While yoga fads come and go, yogis — those who practice yoga regularly — take this ancient discipline seriously. And you should, too. That's because yoga uses a series of carefully executed poses that focus your attention and breathing, as well as stretch your muscles. And the benefits aren't just physical. Studies point to perks for your mind, too.

Keep your memory keen with long-term yoga. When 42 healthy Brazilian senior women agreed to have their brains scanned, researchers discovered something interesting. The 21 women in the group that had practiced yoga for eight years or more had greater thickness in the region of their brains associated with attention and memory — the prefrontal cortex — than the control group that didn't do yoga but maintained a similar level of physical activity.

Why would that matter? It suggests that long-term yoga could change your brain structure in ways that may protect against cognitive decline in old age. How? Researchers think focusing your attention during yoga poses increases activity in the prefrontal cortex.

"In the same way as muscles, the brain develops through training," says Elisa Kozasa, Ph.d., a researcher involved in the study.

Feeling blue? It might be time to strike a pose. Although it's not like a drug in that you can take a pill and call your doctor in the morning, adding the right dosage of yoga could be a helpful intervention for treating depression symptoms.

Adults with major depressive disorder enrolled in a study looking at yoga for depression. One group took three 90-minute yoga classes a week that involved relaxation and breathing exercises in addition to a set number of poses. A second group took two of the same classes weekly. Both groups saw improvements in their depression symptoms, although the group that took three yoga classes a week appeared to benefit the most at the end of the study.

The authors of the study proposed the idea that the mood benefits of yoga and breathing exercises may last about two days before you need your next "dose."

Beyond the mat: 4 ways this no-sweat exercise offers perks at all hours

A great workout for your body also helps strengthen your mind. Research shows exercise like yoga causes your body to create a compound called brain-derived neurotrophic factor (BDNF), which strengthens the connections between your brain cells and even helps new ones grow. But yoga can do more than sharpen your mind — it can help you fend off these troublemakers.

Feeling flexible? Yoga poses protect your heart. High blood pressure is bad news. Not only does it increase your risk of heart attacks, but it can damage your brain, too. There's good news, though. Yoga may help you lower your blood pressure.

In a small study, 80 adults with an irregular heartbeat were divided into two groups. They all underwent standard treatment, but half of the participants were also asked to do yoga involving light movements and deep breathing.

You want to give yoga a try, but the twisty-pretzel movements are too much for you. Try chair yoga instead. In one study, an eight-week program decreased participants' pain and fatigue. And their walking speed improved, too. All accomplished by the seat of their pants. Check YouTube online for free classes.

After 12 weeks, researchers discovered that the people who did yoga had significantly lower blood pressure and heart rates compared with the control group.

Improve your sleep with this simple tip. Tossing and turning all night? You might want to spend some time on the yoga mat. Research shows that regular exercise is linked with a better night's sleep.

A large-scale study conducted by researchers from the Perelman School of Medicine at the University of Pennsylvania examined the sleep and exercise habits of over 429,000 people.

The data revealed that regular exercise — including yoga and pilates — was associated with improved sleep. And that's great for your brain. If you're too tired, it's difficult to concentrate, make decisions, or even remember simple things.

Regular practice beefs up your muscles. Yoga can help keep your body strong and lean as you age. And that's important. As you get older, your muscles can break down and weaken. This process — known as sarcopenia — is linked with dementia.

Recent research published in the *Journal of Aging and Physical Activity* examined how yoga could protect you from getting weaker as you age. Experts compared seven seniors who had been practicing yoga twice a week for at least a year to eight other seniors who rarely exercised.

The study revealed that even though both groups of people had roughly the same body mass index, the yoga group had more muscle, less fat, and better overall balance than the nonexercisers. Researchers think that could be because the yoga group broke down protein in their bodies slower, which helped them maintain more muscle and burn more fat.

Say goodbye to joint pain — yoga soothes arthritis aches. Chronic pain isn't just uncomfortable. Research suggests it can actually weaken your memory. Fortunately, yoga is a natural remedy for arthritis pain.

A recent analysis examined 13 studies about yoga and its effect on arthritis symptoms. Researchers found that this ancient exercise helped improve pain, function, and quality of life in people with arthritis in their knees.

Why is yoga so powerful? It helps strengthen the muscles around your joints which helps improve joint stability and prevent painful arthritis attacks.

"Yoga may be especially well suited to people with arthritis because it combines physical activity with potent stress management and relaxation techniques, and focuses on respecting limitations that can change from day to day," says Dr. Susan J. Bartlett, associate professor at Johns Hopkins School of Medicine in Baltimore.

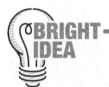
BRIGHT IDEA

Get fit as a fiddle (for free) with SilverSneakers

Think you can't afford to go to the gym? Think again. Many seniors with Medicare Advantage insurance plans have free access to gym memberships and fitness classes that cater to older adults. Dubbed SilverSneakers, the program is available at more than 16,000 locations nationwide.

Yoga is a popular SilverSneakers class, offering a series of seated and standing poses. Instructors provide chairs or large rubber stability balls to help with balance.

Many senior participants believe they gain not only increased flexibility and range of motion, but mental benefits, as well.

Researchers at the Massachusetts Institute of Technology agree. They found in a recent study that SilverSneakers members are more physically active and less isolated or lonely than nonmembers.

The reason? Scientists say the program may cause members to feel more confident and empowered, which in turn increases their sociability.

Visit *silversneakers.com* to find a location near you.

Index